NUTRITION OF THE ELDERLY

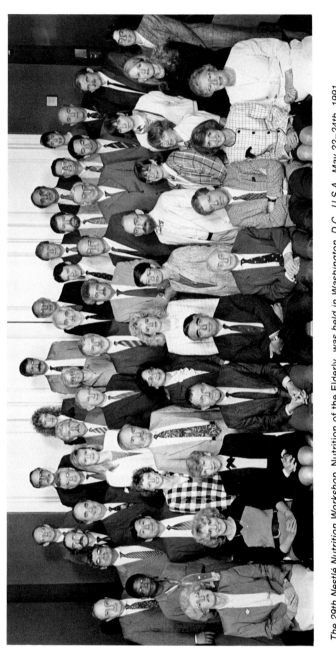

The 29th Nestlé Nutrition Workshop, Nutrition of the Elderly, *was held in Washington, D.C., U.S.A., May 22–24th, 1991.*

Workshop participants (*left to right from first row*): B. Doyle, S. Schiffman, C. N. Meredith, G. Schlierf, P. R. Guesry, H. N. Munro, B. Steen, E. Wedral, L. Davies, G. W. Pla, T. Fujii, A. Kretser, P. Tannen, L. H. Chen, C. Murphy, B. Krouse, D. Rush, R. Ballard-Barbash, D. Porter, M. Parrott, R. Marsden, B. A. Bowman, D. Kritchevsky, R. K. Chandra, J. Baumwoll, M. Podrabsky, P. J. Nestel, H. M. Hodkinson, Z. Glick, W. H. Glinsmann, A. L. de Weck, H. Sato, H. Heseker, Y. Guigoz, N. Melachouris, J. V. G. A. Durnin, W. A. van Staveren, J. A. Edwardson, E. M. Berry, B. Caballero, A. Hüsler, S. S. Schiaffino, R. Clemens, R. Merritt, R. Palubinskas, G. Pace, R. J. Havlik, T. Jackson, A. Reza Kamarei, M. Kealey.

Nestlé Nutrition Workshop Series
Volume 29

NUTRITION OF THE ELDERLY

Editors

Hamish Munro, M.D., F.R.C.P., D.Sc.
Senior Scientist
Agricultural Research Service
United States Department of Agriculture
Human Nutrition Research Center
on Aging at Tufts
Boston, Massachusetts, USA

Günter Schlierf, M.D.
Professor of Medicine and Geriatrics
Bethanien Hospital
Heidelberg, Germany

NESTLÉ NUTRITION SERVICES

RAVEN PRESS ■ NEW YORK

Nestec Ltd., 55 Avenue Nestlé, CH-1800 Vevey, Switzerland
Raven Press, Ltd., 1185 Avenue of the Americas, New York,
New York 10036

Made in the United States of America

Library of Congress Cataloging-in-Publication Data
Nutrition of the elderly / editors, Hamish Munro, Günter Schlierf.
     p.   cm.—(Nestlé Nutrition workshop series ; v. 29)
    Proceedings of the 29th Nestlé Nutrition
Workshop on "Nutrition of the Elderly," held in Washington, D.C.,
May 22–24, 1991.
    Includes bibliographical references and index.
    ISBN 0-88167-874-0
    1. Nutrition disorders in old age—Congresses. 2. Aged—
Nutrition—Congresses. 3. Alzheimer's disease—Nutritional
aspects—Congresses. 4. Osteoporosis—Nutritional aspects—
Congresses. I. Munro, Hamish N. (Hamish Nisbet) II. Schlierf,
Günter. III. Nestlé Nutrition Workshop on "Nutrition of the
Elderly" (1991 : Washington, D.C.) IV. Series.
    [DNLM: 1. Aging—physiology—congresses. 2. Alzheimer's
Disease—prevention & control—congresses. 3. Nutrition—in old age—
congresses. 4. Osteoporosis—prevention & control—congresses.
W1 NE228 v.29]
RC620.6.N88 1992
613.2'084'6—dc20
DNLM/DLC
for Library of Congress   91-40901

9 8 7 6 5 4 3 2 1

Preface

In many advanced countries, the proportion of people 65 years and older has grown to 12% to 16% of the population. For example, at the beginning of this century, old people accounted for 4% of Americans, whereas at the end of this century it is anticipated that they will represent 14% of the population. This imposes a heavy burden on the health care system. In recent years, increasing interest has been paid to the role nutrition has played in promoting and sustaining the health and function of our senior citizens.

This Workshop brought together an impressive group of investigators who have contributed to our understanding of the relationship between nutrition and the aging process, as well as the nutrient needs of people who have attained senior citizenship. This volume begins with sociology, namely the health statistics and eating habits of old people, and is followed by an assessment of physiological changes that occur during aging. It is succeeded by an account of the specific nutrient needs of the elderly. Several chapters follow on the role nutritional factors play in selected diseases expressed in older people, namely osteoporosis and Alzheimer's disease. Finally, practical aspects of the nutrition of the elderly at home or in institutions are described.

This volume presents a refreshing collection of essays on various aspects of nutrition in relation to aging, each followed by a lively discussion. It is hoped that these new insights will stimulate more work on the relationship of nutritional status and nutrient intakes to optimal aging.

HAMISH MUNRO, M.D., F.R.C.P., D.Sc.
Boston, Massachusetts, USA

"There is nothing better for a man than that he should eat and drink and that his soul should enjoy good in his labor" (Ecclesiastes 2, 24). Most would agree with the Bible that good food and fair work rank high in the pleasures of men and women.

There are good reasons why eating and drinking should be of particular importance to the elderly. Indeed, the quality and quantity of life are markedly affected by adequate nutrition. Many disorders which are prevalent in the elderly have their roots in poor nutritional habits. For example, there are diseases from overconsumption such as diabetes and atherosclerosis, and also from insufficient nutrient supply such as osteoporosis and goiter. A healthy diet before we become old, and sufficient nourishment when we are old and sick, are matters of high priority.

v

In this Workshop, these topics have been identified and discussed, and I hope that the results of the Workshop will have an impact on the theory and practice of nutrition in the elderly.

GÜNTER SCHLIERF, M.D.
Heidelberg, Germany

Foreword

The rapid increase in life expectancy in industrialized countries, over the last century has been due almost entirely to the cure, or prevention, of disease through the development of new drugs, techniques, or immunization. Modern society has been left with a socioeconomic problem that has become acute over the last 20 years—the millions of institutionalized elderly.

Although lengthening the human life span is laudable, if the result is that numerous old people have to live in institutions for decades, in bad health, with physical and intellectual limitations preventing them from enjoying the extra years modern medicine has granted them, then I believe that we have only fulfilled part of our duty.

We need to act quickly to catch up on the problem of these unfulfilling extra years of life. The first priority for the future is not so much to increase life expectancy, but rather to improve the general well-being and health status of elderly people in such a way that they can fully enjoy a longer life with not only physical, but also intellectual, independence.

In order to achieve this goal, the *leitmotif* must be prevention. For example, we know that it is much easier to prevent osteoporosis than to cure it. The same can certainly be said for muscular atrophy, probably for the immunodepression of aging, and maybe even for Alzheimer's disease.

Prevention, to be fully effective, should start as soon as possible after 50 years of age. The prevention program should include eating a wide variety of foods, physical activity, intellectual training, moderation in the use of tobacco, alcohol, and saturated fats, and a regular intake of vitamins, trace minerals, long chain polyunsaturated fatty acids, natural antioxidants, and so on, in a way which is enjoyable enough to ensure long-term compliance. People who adopt with pleasure such a program would not only enjoy a longer active life, but, as a fringe benefit, should also get closer to their genetically-programmed biological age limit of 100 years and more.

We wanted to explore the various hypotheses behind this challenging program, and the 29th Nestlé Nutrition Workshop on "Nutrition of the Elderly" (which as it turned out could perhaps have been better called "Preventive Nutrition") gave us exciting opportunities to confirm our enthusiasm about achieving a brighter future.

PIERRE R. GUESRY, M.D.
Vice President, Nestec Ltd.
Vevey, Switzerland

Contents

Practical Aspects of Nutrition of the Elderly

Contributors

Elliot M. Berry
Department of Medicine
Hadassah University Hospital
P.O. Box 12000
il-91120 Jerusalem, Israel

Jean-Philippe Bonjour
Department of Medicine
Division of Clinical Pathophysiology
University Hospital of Geneva
24 Rue Micheli-du-Crest
1211 Geneva 4, Switzerland

Barbara A. Bowman
Department of Nutrition and Dietetics
Georgia State University
University Plaza
Atlanta, Georgia 30303-3083, USA

Louise Davies
Gerontology Nutrition
Royal Free Hospital School of Medicine
Rowland Hill Street
London NW3 2QE, England, UK

Alain L. de Weck
Institute of Clinical Immunology
Inselspital
3010 Bern, Switzerland

John V. G. A. Durnin
Institute of Physiology
University of Glasgow
Glasgow G12 8QQ, Scotland, UK

James A. Edwardson
Medical Research Council
Neurochemical Pathology Unit
Newcastle General Hospital
Westgate Road
Newcastle-upon-Tyne NE4 6BE,
England, UK

Zvi Glick
UCLA School of Medicine
Department of Veterans Affairs
Sepulveda Medical Center
GRECC (11E)
16111 Plummer Street
Sepulveda, California 91343, USA

Richard J. Havlik
Epidemiology, Demography and
  Biometry Program
National Institute on Aging
National Institutes of Health
7201 Wisconsin Avenue
Bethesda, Maryland 20892, USA

Helmut Heseker
Institut für Ernährungswissenschaft
der Justus-Liebig-Universität Giessen
Goethestrasse 55
6300 Giessen, Germany

H. Malcolm Hodkinson
Department of Geriatric Medicine
University College London
St. Pancras Hospital
4 St. Pancras Way
London NW1 0PE, England, UK

David Kritchevsky
The Wistar Institute
3601 Spruce Street
Philadelphia, Pennsylvania 19104, USA

Werner Kübler
Institut für Ernährungswissenschaft
der Justus-Liebig-Universität Giessen
Goethestrasse 55
6300 Giessen, Germany

Robert Lindsay
Regional Bone Center
Helen Hayes Hospital
Route 9W
West Haverstraw, New York, 10993,
USA

Carol N. Meredith
Division of Clinical Nutrition
School of Medicine
University of California at Davis
Davis, California 95616, USA

Walter Mertz
Beltsville Human Nutrition Research
 Center
Agricultural Research Service
USDA
Beltsville, Maryland 20705, USA

Pierre J. Meunier
INSERM, Unité 234,
Service de Rhumatologie et de
 Pathologie Osseuse
Hôpital Edouard Herriot
69437 Lyon Cédex 03, France

Hamish N. Munro
USDA
ARS, Human Nutrition Research Center
 on Aging
711 Washington Street
Boston, Massachusetts 02111, USA

Claire Murphy
University of California, San Diego
 Medical Center,
Department of Psychology
San Diego State University
6363 Alvarado Court
San Diego, California 92120, USA

Paul J. Nestel
CSIRO
Division of Human Nutrition
P.O. Box 10041
Gouger Street
Adelaide, South Australia 5000,
 Australia

Hiroshi Sato
The Second Department of Internal
 Medicine
Tohoku University School of Medicine
1-1 Seiryo-cho, Aoba-Ku
Sendai 980, Japan

Susan Schiffman
Department of Psychology
Duke University
Durham, North Carolina 27706, USA

Günter Schlierf
Department of Medicine/Geriatrics
Bethanien Hospital Heidelberg
Rohrbacher Strasse 149
6900 Heidelberg 1, Germany

Bertil Steen
Department of Geriatrics and Long-
 Term Care Medicine
Gothenburg University
Vasa Hospital
41133 Gothenburg, Sweden

Wija A. van Staveren
Department of Human Nutrition
Wageningen Agricultural University
Bomenweg 2
6700 EV Wageningen, The Netherlands

Bruno Vellas
Centre Hospitalo-Universitaire de
 Toulouse
Hôpital Purpan
Place Dr. Baylac
31300 Toulouse, France

Invited Attendees

Rachel Ballard-Barbash / Washington,
 DC, USA
Joel Baumwoll / New York, New
 York, USA
Ann Bell / Washington, DC, USA
Alexis Brown / Washington, DC,
 USA

Benjamin Caballero / Baltimore,
 Maryland, USA
R. K. Chandra / Newfoundland,
 Canada
Linda H. Chen / Lexington,
 Kentucky, USA

Bridget Doyle / *Columbia, Missouri, USA*

Sandra B. Eskin / *Washington, DC, USA*

Walter H. Glinsmann / *Washington, DC, USA*

Judith Hallfrisch / *Baltimore, Maryland, USA*

Jennifer Harper / *Solon, Ohio, USA*

Tamara Harris / *Hyattsville, Maryland, USA*

Linda Jackson / *Washington, DC, USA*

A. Reza Kamarei / *Deerfield, Illinois, USA*

Marta Kealey / *Alexandria, Virginia, USA*

Fritz Kessinger / *Washington, DC, USA*

Alison Kretser / *New Milford, Connecticut, USA*

Barbara Krouse / *Solon, Ohio, USA*

John Leonard / *Washington, DC, USA*

J. Michael McGinnis / *Washington, DC, USA*

Ruth Marsden / *Alexandria, Virginia, USA*

Mary Rose Oakar / *Washington, DC, USA*

Gary W. Pace / *Deerfield, Illinois, USA*

Marian Parrott / *Washington, DC, USA*

Mark Paskowsky / *Washington, DC, USA*

Gwendolyn W. Pla / *Washington, DC, USA*

Mary Podrabsky / *Grand Rapids, Michigan, USA*

Donna Porter / *Washington, DC, USA*

David Rush / *Boston, Massachusetts, USA*

Margaret A. Schaaf / *Boston, Massachusetts, USA*

S. Stephen Schiaffino / *Bethesda, Maryland, USA*

Marta Sotomayor / *Washington, DC, USA*

Peter Tannen / *New York, New York, USA*

Janet E. Tenney / *Washington, DC, USA*

Juanita Yates / *Washington, DC, USA*

Nestlé Participants

Roger A. Clemens, *Nestlé Food Company, Glendale, California, USA*

Tim Crull, *Nestlé USA Inc., Washington, DC, USA*

Takato Fujii, *Nestlé K. K., Tokyo, Japan*

Pierre R. Guesry, *Nestec Ltd., Vevey, Switzerland*

Yves Guigoz, *Nestlé Research Center, Lausanne, Switzerland*

Jennifer Harper, *Stouffer Foods, Solon, Ohio, USA*

Angelo Hüsler, *Nestec Ltd., Vevey, Switzerland*

Thad Jackson, *Nestlé USA Inc., Washington, DC, USA*

Barbara Krouse, *Stouffer Foods, Solon, Ohio, USA*

Nicholas Melachouris, *Westreco Inc., Van Nuys, California, USA*

Russell Merritt, *Nestlé Food Company, Glendale, California, USA*

Rita Palubinskas, *Stouffer Foods, Solon, Ohio, USA*

Elaine Wedral, *Westreco, Inc., New Milford, Connecticut, USA*

Nestlé Nutrition Workshop Series

Nutrition of the Elderly, edited by H. Munro and
G. Schlierf, Nestlé Nutrition Workshop Series, Vol. 29,
Nestec Ltd., Vevey/Raven Press, Ltd., New York 1992.

Nutrition of the Elderly: Introduction

Hamish N. Munro

*USDA Human Nutrition Research Center on Aging at Tufts,
Boston, Massachusetts 02111, USA*

At the beginning of this century, only 4% of the population of the United States was over 65 years of age. By 1976 this proportion had risen to 11% and is projected to attain 14% by the year 2000 (1). This is important because senior citizens make disproportionate demands on health care. An interesting study in Massachusetts emphasizes the extent of the needs of senior citizens for health care as they age (2). The authors compute the number of years an elderly person is likely to live independently and the number of subsequent years he or she will need assistance in rising from bed, washing, dressing, and/or eating. Thus, for persons aged 65 to 69 years, it is computed that independent living will continue for an average of 9.3 years for men and 10.6 years for women. This is followed by 3.8 years of dependent living for men and 8.9 years for women. One can speculate that independent living is determined by the continued adequacy of the neuromuscular system, and that loss of this occurs at the same rate in both men and women, whereas longer survival of women in a dependent state may reflect their slower development of lethal cardiovascular diseases.

Nutrition has been recognized only recently as an important factor influencing the functional outcome of aging. In the course of the symposium, it will become evident that nutrients consumed during earlier adult life as well as in the later years can affect the terminal years of the life span. To provide some order while analyzing the evidence of dietary involvement in the aging process, we can assemble the data in several categories. First, changes in body composition and in organ function occur throughout adult life, making old age the recipient of adverse processes begun at earlier ages (e.g., loss of bone density leading to osteoporosis and fracture). Second, many degenerative diseases first assert themselves in middle life and persist into old age (e.g., cardiovascular diseases). Nutritional habits are prime factors in the etiology of some of these diseases. Third, the amounts of many individual dietary nutrients needed to maintain optimal health in old age still require quantification. This is important because the elderly tend to consume less food (3).

This conference emphasizes factors underlying nutrient needs for the elderly. The present workshop provides a wide range of topics relevant to nutrition and aging and to old age. It includes the sociology of aging, an extensive account of physiological changes as aging progresses, specific nutrient needs of the elderly, the relevance of some age-related diseases, and finally practical aspects of the nutritional state of the elderly. In addition to this workshop, recent books (e.g., 4,5) on nutrition of the elderly provide further information.

AGE-RELATED BODILY CHANGES

Throughout adult life, there are continuous changes in body composition, in tissue function, and in metabolism. Thus, lean body mass is progressively reduced as age advances, whereas fat accumulates (6). The loss of lean body mass is most extensive from skeletal muscle, as demonstrated by the large reduction in urinary output of muscle-derived creatinine and 3-methylhistidine by the elderly (7). Along with the changes in body composition goes reduced muscle function, as illustrated by decreasing muscle strength, which can be demonstrated by measuring hand grip of men and women of various ages (8). Shock has assembled the effects of aging on the function of various organs by plotting their residual capacity at different ages (8). As measured on men aged 80 years compared with those of 30 years, loss of function was found to vary from 50% reduction of renal blood flow to only 15% for nerve conduction. Little of this has been attributed to the diet of humans. The most dramatic effect of diet on aging is, however, provided by the numerous studies on rats subjected to partial food restriction, which results in longer survival of these animals accompanied by delayed loss of tissue function (9).

CHRONIC DISEASES IN RELATION TO NUTRITION

Much literature has appeared in which components of the diet can be linked to the appearance of specific diseases in middle and later life. Several reports have emerged, the most recent being the Diet and Health Report of the National Academy of Sciences (10) and the Surgeon General's Report (11). Both of these summarize cautiously the evidence relating long-term patterns of dietary intake to the frequency of chronic diseases in later adult life. Some major chronic diseases are probably influenced by long-term intake of fat, calcium, sodium, vitamin A, or fiber; the diseases involved are atherosclerosis, coronary heart disease, hypertension, osteoporosis, diseases of immune function, and so forth. These relationships will be evaluated in this workshop.

There is still debate about the ideal body weight for adults of various ages. In a recent commentary, Willett *et al.* (12) challenged the proposal of the Dietary Guidelines for Americans, which suggests that adults over 35 years of age can substantially raise the body weight recommended for longest survival. Instead, Willett *et al.* produced arguments that ideal body weight does not change during adult life.

NUTRIENT NEEDS AND INTAKES OF ELDERLY PEOPLE

Our knowledge of the nutrient requirements of elderly people remains inadequately documented. The National Academy of Sciences' Recommended Dietary Allowances (13) provide for only three age-related categories for adults, namely, 19 to 24 years, 25 to 50 years, and 51+ years. The latter represents the age range from 51 years up to and beyond 100 years. Better knowledge of the effects of aging on nutritional status over this wide range is restricted by the lack of available data such as the limitation of the HANES surveys of representative US populations to persons not exceeding 74 years of age. In contrast, we need to be able to establish the dietary allowances for a 90-year-old man in a nursing home consuming 1250 kcal per day, compared with a middle-aged man eating 2500 kcal per day and presumably consuming twice the protein, vitamin, and mineral intakes of the 90-year-old man. Does this large reduction in nutrient intake result in impaired function and survival? If the elderly are considered to require the same minimum amounts as do younger adults, then the voluntary low intakes of old people may risk deficiency. Detailed analysis of the literature on the nutrient needs of the elderly is provided by this workshop and is also documented elsewhere (4).

Regarding the frequency of inadequate intakes by the elderly and the occurrence of clinically diagnosable evidence of deficiency, the literature has to be approached with caution. For example, the blood levels of selected vitamins can be compared in free-living and in nursing home elderly in two locations, namely, Northern Ireland (14) and New Jersey (15). In Northern Ireland (Table 1), subnormal thiamin levels were just as infrequent in nursing home elderly as in free-living elderly, whereas in New Jersey there were many more subnormal thiamin values in the blood of the free-living population. In the case of vitamin B_6, subnormal levels were much more frequent among the nursing-home elderly in both locations, whereas subnormal blood values for vitamin C were more frequent in the nursing home elderly of Northern Ireland but were much fewer in the nursing home population than in the free-living elderly in New Jersey. These distributions probably reflect differences in the pattern of vitamin intakes at the two locations. More important is the need for evidence of

TABLE 1. *Percentage of subnormal values for three vitamins in the blood of elderly subjects in Northern Ireland (14) and in New Jersey (15) who were either free-living or in nursing homes*

Population	Thiamin	Vitamin B_6	Vitamin C
Northern Ireland			
Free-living	13	43	23
Nursing home	11	63	56
New Jersey			
Free-living	25	18	24
Nursing home	4	37	4

clinical deficiency in elderly people associated with such subnormal values and, finally, whether these levels impair bodily function and survival.

In this context, it is worth comparing two studies of the nutritional status of elderly adults. One was made on a group of British elderly people who were representative of the British population and included elderly people with chronic wasting diseases (16). The other was a Boston population of elderly people who had been purged of subjects suffering from debilitating diseases (17). The British survey evaluated 365 men and women 70 years and older and included measures of nutrient intake, biochemical tests of deficiency, and clinical evaluation. The survey identified malnutrition in 26 subjects. For subjects not yet 80 years old, the frequencies were less (6% men, 5% women) than for those 80 years and older (12% men, 8% women). Protein-energy malnutrition was the most common deficiency. All but 1 of the 26 malnourished subjects had long-term debilitating conditions such as chronic bronchitis, emphysema, mental depression, and so forth. These subjects showed a smaller intake of nutrients than the other elderly persons who had no evidence of malnutrition. The Boston study (17) excluded those elderly people having diseases associated with wasting and was rewarded by the absence of overt malnutrition in the remaining subjects.

FACTORS AFFECTING NUTRITIONAL STATUS OF THE ELDERLY

In view of the above demonstration of severe malnutrition secondary to certain diseases, there are other factors listed by Exton-Smith (18) that tend to put the elderly at risk of malnutrition. First, the environment may provide adverse nutritional conditions. These include poverty, which may restrict food choices. This also occurs in cases of house-bound elderly people. Loss of interest in food can occur and this is sometimes reversed by communal eating. Ignorance of the basic principles of adequate nutrition can lead to unbalanced nutrient intake, especially in the case of widowed men who have never cooked a meal.

Second, malnutrition can be secondary to pathological factors. In addition to the conditions identified in the British survey described above, malnutrition can also be associated with gastrointestinal features of aging such as achlorhydria, malabsorption following gastrectomy, as well as inefficient mastication from ill-fitting dentures and the use of certain drugs interacting with utilization of specific nutrients.

In conclusion, it must be recognized that the nutritional status of the elderly is subject to more adverse environmental factors than occur in the case of the young. More study is needed of the interaction of nutrients with the preservation of function in the elderly, and procedures for screening the elderly for malnutrition (19) should be extended (5).

REFERENCES

1. Brody JB, Brock DB. Epidemiological and statistical characteristics of the United States elderly population. In: Finch CE, Schneider EL, eds. *Handbook of biology of aging*. 2nd ed. New York: Van Nostrand Rheinhold, 1985: 3–26.

2. Katz S, Branch LG, Branson MH, Papsidero JH, Beck JC, Greer DS. Active life expectancy. *N Engl J Med* 1983;309:1212–24.
3. McGandy RB, Barrows CH, Spanias A, Meredith A, Stone JL, Norris AH. Nutrient intakes and energy expenditure in men of different ages. *J Gerontol* 1966;21:581–7.
4. Munro HN, Danford DE, eds. *Nutrition, aging and the elderly*. New York: Plenum Press, 1989.
5. Armbrecht HJ, Prendergast JM, Coe RM, eds. *Nutritional intervention in the aging process*. New York: Springer–Verlag, 1984: 1–343.
6. Cohn SH, Vartsky D, Yasumura S, *et al.* Compartmental body composition based on total body nitrogen, potassium and calcium. *Am J Physiol* 1980;239:E524–30.
7. Uauy R, Winterer JC, Bilmazes C, *et al.* The changing pattern of whole body protein metabolism in aging humans. *J Gerontol* 1978;33:663–71.
8. Shock NW. Energy metabolism, caloric intake and physical activity of the aging. In: Carlson LA, ed. *Nutrition in old age*. Uppsala: Wiksel, 1972:12–23.
9. Masoro EJ. Nutrition and aging in animal models. In: Munro HN, Danford DE, eds. *Human nutrition: a comprehensive treatise*, vol 6, *Nutrition, aging, and the elderly*. New York: Plenum, 1989:25–41.
10. National Research Council. *Diet and health: implications for reducing chronic disease risk*. Washington, DC: National Academy Press, 1989.
11. The Surgeon General's Report. Nutrition and Health. Chapter 16, Aging. Washington, DC: US Dept of Health and Human Services, Publication No. 88:50210, 1988:595–627.
12. Willett WC, Stampfer M, Manson J, Van Itallie T. New weight guidelines for Americans: justified or injudicious. *Am J Clin Nutr* 1991;53:1102–3.
13. National Research Council. *Recommended dietary allowances*. 10th ed. Washington, DC: National Academy Press, 1989.
14. Vir SC, Love AHG. Nutritional status of institutionalized and non-institutionalized aged in Belfast, Northern Ireland. *Am J Clin Nutr* 1979;32:1934–47.
15. Baker H, Frank O, Thind IS, Jaslow SP, Louria DB. Vitamin profiles in elderly persons living at home or in nursing homes versus profiles in healthy young subjects. *J Am Geriatr Soc* 1979;29: 444–50.
16. Dept of Health and Social Security. *A nutrition survey of the elderly*. Reports on Health and Social Subjects, No 16. London: Her Majesty's Stationery Office, 1979.
17. McGandy RB, Russell RM, Hartz SC, *et al.* Nutritional status survey of healthy non-institutionalized elderly: nutrient intakes from three-day diet records and nutrient supplements. *Nutr Res* 1986;6: 785–98.
18. Exton-Smith AN. Nutritional status: diagnosis and prevention of malnutrition. In: Exton-Smith AN, Caird FI, eds. *Metabolic and nutritional disorders in the elderly*. Bristol: Wright, 1980:66–76.
19. Munro HN, McGandy RB, Hartz SC, Russell RM, Jacob RA, Otradovec CL. Protein nutriture of group of free-living elderly. *Am J Clin Nutr* 1987;46:586–92.

Nutrition of the Elderly, edited by H. Munro and
G. Schlierf, Nestlé Nutrition Workshop Series, Vol. 29,
Nestec Ltd., Vevey/Raven Press, Ltd., New York 1992.

Health Statistics on Older Persons

Richard J. Havlik

*National Institute on Aging, National Institutes of Health,
Bethesda, Maryland 20892, USA*

In considering nutritional issues in older persons, an awareness of the demographic trends toward an aging population and of the common conditions and diseases in this subgroup is essential. This chapter will focus on health statistics rather than on nutritional relationships; however, many of the diseases and conditions to which elderly people are prone will have a nutritional component, either as a possible cause or as a result of the presence of the condition.

An important area in aging research, not addressed directly by health statistics, is the potential relationship of nutrition to the usual aging processes themselves. At least theoretically, it is important to attempt to differentiate the adverse effects of increasing age from the effects of chronic diseases, many of which increase at older ages (1). If this could be accomplished, then the goals of a nutrition program might be defined both in terms of a beneficial effect on aging processes and in terms of prevention or treatment of nutritionally related chronic diseases.

Relevant information on vital statistics, health status, nutrition, and use of health services among older persons in the United States is collected by the National Center for Health Statistics (NCHS) through various data systems, and includes mortality statistics, the Hospital Discharge Survey, the Health Interview Survey, the National Health and Nutrition Examination Survey, and the Nursing Home Survey (2).

DEMOGRAPHIC IMPERATIVE

In 1985, according to the Bureau of the Census, about 12% of the total US population was 65 years and over and about 3 million, or 1%, was 85 years and over (2). Because of the "baby boom" there are projections for major increases in the older populations in the 21st century. In the United States the estimated increase is from the current 30 million to about 55 million older persons in 2030 (3). If the decreases in mortality have been underestimated, the number could be greater. This has raised some concerns about the ability of various social security and hospital trust funds to meet future needs. Similar population projections have been made for both developed and developing countries (4).

DEATHS BY CAUSE

In 1987, about 70% of deaths, or 1.5 million, occurred among those 65 years and over (5). Although the absolute numbers were among the highest in US history, when adjusted for the larger numbers of older persons the rates were among the lowest. Heart, cancer, and stroke deaths form the great majority, with lung disease, diabetes, accidents, and infections making up the remainder (Table 1). Alzheimer's disease does not appear on the list, possibly because of underreporting in mortality statistics. Nutrition may play a role in certain aspects of these deaths; for example, through effects of cardiovascular risk factors on heart disease, fat and fiber on cancer, obesity on diabetes, and infections resulting in poor nutrition. Because of the heterogeneity in health status among older persons, it is important to examine subgroups. For example, at younger ages death rates are higher in black than in white women; however, there is an apparent crossover between the races at older ages, with black women having lower death rates. This phenomenon may represent survival of a selected and less disease-prone subgroup of older blacks (6).

In multiple cause-of-death listings (which include all information on death certificates), heart disease increases in death certificate entries from 40% to more than half. However, diabetes becomes much more common as a reason for death than when only the underlying cause is used. Even with these changes, the numerical ranking of each cause remains about the same as when only the underlying cause is listed (7). In terms of long-term mortality trends, for all ages including the oldest ages and for both major race groups, death rates, especially for cardiovascular diseases, have decreased over the last 20 years; however, during this period coronary

TABLE 1. *Deaths and death rates for the 10 leading causes of death in persons aged 65 years and over, United States, 1987*

Rank order	Cause of death	Number	Rate (per 100,000)
	All causes	1,509,686	5059.9
1	Diseases of heart	618,989	2074.6
2	Malignant neoplasms including neoplasms of lymphatic and hematopoietic tissues	316,199	1059.8
3	Cerebrovascular diseases	129,784	435.0
4	Chronic obstructive pulmonary disease	64,451	216.0
5	Pneumonia and influenza	60,542	202.9
6	Diabetes mellitus	28,377	95.1
7	Accidents and adverse effects	25,838	86.6
	All other accidents and adverse effects	6,781	22.7
	Motor vehicle accidents	19,057	63.9
8	Atherosclerosis	21,372	71.6
9	Nephritis, nephrotic syndrome, and nephrosis	18,249	61.2
10	Septicemia	15,868	53.2
	All other causes residual	210,017	703.9

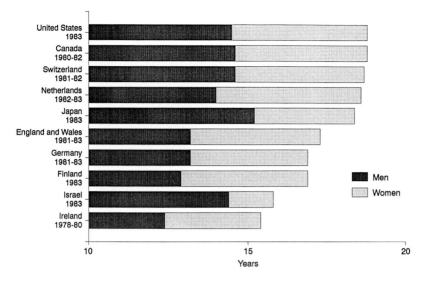

FIG. 1. Life expectancy at age 65 in selected countries.

heart disease mortality has decreased by almost 40% in the United States. Since the decline occurred at older as well as at younger ages, some have attributed it to improved medical care, but nutritional changes may have accounted for part of the decline, through a beneficial effect on cardiovascular risk factors. Although Japan has the longest life expectancy at birth, from the age of 65 years life expectancy becomes longer among persons in other selected countries (8). However, life expectancy for women is always higher than for men in the developed countries (Fig. 1).

HOSPITAL DISCHARGES

Cross-sectional data for 1984 are available from the US National Hospital Discharge Survey (Fig. 2) (9). They show higher discharge rates at older ages. For men (not shown), diseases of heart and the other major causes of death (cancer and stroke) are also the major causes of hospital admissions. In the oldest group stroke surpasses cancer. Hyperplasia of the prostate is a relatively frequent cause as well. In a comparable analysis of hospital discharges for women, a similar relationship was present (Fig. 2). Importantly, the second major cause among the oldest group of women was fractures—most of which were fractures of the hip. These were likely to have been secondary to underlying osteoporosis (possibly related to inadequate calcium intake) and to falls precipitating the fracture. Nutritionally related diabetes also becomes an important cause for hospital admission in older women.

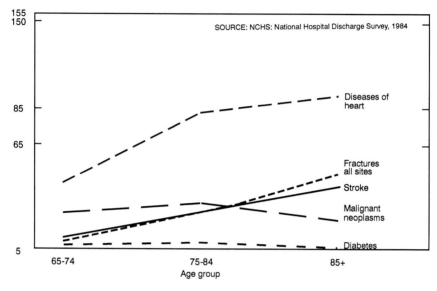

FIG. 2. Diagnosis of hospital discharges in US women by age group in 1984 (per 1,000 population).

CORONARY RISK FACTORS

Health examination estimates of the frequency of definite hypertension in the United States (defined as a blood pressure of 160 mm Hg systolic, 95 diastolic, or currently receiving treatment) are shown in Table 2 (10). The rates for men are in the range of 40% to 50%, depending on race, but higher (40–70%) for women. More than 75% of black women 65 years of age or older have definite hypertension. Blood

TABLE 2. *Americans age 55 years and over living in communities with risk factors, 1976–1980*

Race–sex–age subgroup	Definite hypertension (%)	High-risk serum cholesterol (%)	Overweight (%)
White men			
55–64	38.0	18.6	28.6
65 and over	43.6	13.7	25.8
Black men			
55–64	53.9	16.7	26.0
65 and over	45.2	12.1	26.4
White women			
55–64	38.8	30.6	34.8
65 and over	53.4	29.9	36.5
Black women			
55–64	61.7	29.7	59.4
65 and over	76.5	25.0	60.8

Source: NCHS: National Health and Nutrition Examination Survey II, 1976–1980.

cholesterol levels have tended to decrease over the past 20 years. During this period, there has been a cholesterol decrease of about 6 to 8 mg per deciliter, which is evident in both older men and women (11). High-risk serum cholesterol is defined according to the NIH Consensus Conference cut point (serum level of 268 mg per deciliter). Although about 15% of men are at high risk, women are twice as high at 30%. Since cholesterol continues to increase with age in older women, this may be the reason for the higher percentage at risk. An arbitrary definition of overweight uses as an ideal the weight distribution of younger men and women. The Quetelet index for the upper 15% is defined as the standard. Using this definition, about 60% of older black women are overweight. The frequency of overweight is certainly high enough to suggest that an overnutrition problem exists in this subgroup.

HEALTH STATUS

The National Health Interview Survey is a household survey; Table 3 presents a compilation of selected data on self-reported physician-diagnosed diseases for 3 years (1982–1984) (12). At age 65 years and over it appears that there is a slightly higher percentage of whites with chronic bronchitis than blacks. The hypertension figures and relationships are comparable to those from examinations. For diabetes, the percentages for both black men and women are about twice those for whites. This is predominately non–insulin-dependent diabetes. The frequency of arthritis is higher for the 65 years old and over subgroup compared to those of 55 to 64 years. About two-thirds of black women report arthritis.

Reported symptoms of urinary incontinence are greater for women than men. They increase with age from about 6% to 15% at the oldest ages (13). Hearing impairment

TABLE 3. *Americans age 55 years and over living in communities*

Race–sex–age subgroup	Chronic bronchitis (%)	Hypertension (%)	Diabetes (%)	Arthritis (%)
White men				
55–64	4.2	28.6	6.4	28.0
65 and over	5.3	31.7	8.0	39.2
Black men				
55–64	4.6[a]	36.5	15.3	28.3
65 and over	1.6[a]	37.1	12.1	46.8
White women				
55–64	5.6	30.1	6.3	41.3
65 and over	6.7	42.9	8.5	54.0
Black women				
55–64	7.9	50.4	14.9	47.1
65 and over	3.6[a]	64.3	21.1	64.0

Source: NCHS: National Health Interview Survey, 1982–1984.
[a] Indicates large standard error.

is defined as the reported presence of deafness in one or both ears or the presence of any other trouble with hearing. Depending on age, from 30.1% to 58.2% of men reported a hearing impairment compared to between 17.6% and 48.4% of women, an obvious excess in the men (14). The category of visual impairment, which combines reported blindness in one or both eyes and any other trouble in seeing, was found less frequently than hearing impairment in from 9.4% to 28.5% in the oldest subgroup. The frequency of visual impairments was similar in men and women; however, there was a significant excess of reported cataracts in women when compared with men (14).

LIMITATIONS IN ACTIVITIES

In a US survey of non-institutionalized older persons, questions about the basic activities of daily living (ADLs) were asked (15). Almost 20% indicated some difficulty walking, with lesser frequencies of the more serious impairments such as difficulty moving about or eating. In a similar analysis limited to those 85 years and older, about 40% of women had difficulty walking (2). Visual and hearing impairments, besides limiting communication and sensory stimulation, may also contribute to compromising the physical mobility and independent activity of the elderly.

For the non-institutionalized older persons, various community services have become available to provide both social and medical support. About 10% ate at least one meal at a "senior center" and a smaller percentage received "meals on wheels." As might have been anticipated, those living alone used the senior center and meal service more frequently (16).

NURSING HOME RESIDENTS

Of the 30 million persons 65 years and over in 1985, 4.6%, or 1,300,000, resided in nursing homes. For the subgroup 85 years and over, 20% were resident in a nursing home. These data come from the National Nursing Home Survey (17). When compared with 1977, a higher proportion of nursing home residents had difficulties with ADLs and presumably were sicker in 1985. There are projections that 43% of Americans who turn 65 will spend some time in a nursing home at a point in the remainder of their lives (18).

VITALITY

The opposite end of the spectrum from nursing home residents is represented by persons with physical, social, and mental vitality or those exhibiting "successful aging" (19). Questions about regular exercise and other activities were asked during a survey directed to older individuals living at home. From other surveys it is known that such exercise includes walking, gardening, and perhaps light calisthenics, but does not include many vigorous activities such as marathon running. At all the older ages except perhaps in the oldest women, there was a subgroup of about 25% that reported exercising regularly (20).

Measures of social support have been used in epidemiologic studies as variables that predict a favorable mortality or morbidity outcome. However, such measures can be used as indicators of social vitality. They should suggest potentially active family and social relationships or activities. For example, during a 2-week period more than 80% to 86% of older persons talked by phone with a relative or friend and more than 70% saw a friend or relative (20). Also, about 50% attended church or synagogue or related activity and about 25% went to a show or movie, sports event, club meeting, classes, or other group events. Of course, active leadership rather than passive participation should be assessed to determine social vitality.

The CES-D (Center for Epidemiologic Studies-Depression) scale questions have been used to address mental vitality (21). The scale consists of 20 questions about being "blue, sad, and having crying spells"; however, four of the items are positive factors rather than negative ones. "Happy, good as others, enjoy life, and hopeful about the future" are asked in the context of frequency during the past week. In older persons 50% to 63% reported positive feelings for 5 to 7 days per week (20). Men were generally more positive than women. When compared to the younger subgroups, such attitudes were comparable in both age subgroups.

The identification of nutritional or other factors that might promote vitality as well as prevent diseases is a challenging area for research. A goal suggested by Dr. Fries is the elimination of premature mortality with both deaths and morbidity being compressed or clustered at the oldest age biologically possible (22). In summary, one of the outcomes of nutritional research should be prevention of chronic diseases and disability that force nursing home admissions or minimize vitality. Such a result would contribute greatly to "successful aging" becoming more common among older people in the United States and elsewhere.

REFERENCES

1. Schneider EL, Reed JD. Modulations of aging processes. In: Finch CE, Schneider EL, eds. *Handbook of the biology of aging*. New York: Van Nostrand Reinhold Co, 1985:45–76.
2. National Center for Health Statistics, Havlik RJ, Liu BM, Kovar MG, *et al*. Health statistics on older persons, United States, 1986. *Vital and health statistics*. Series 3, No 25. DHHS Publication No (PHS) 87-1409. Washington, DC: US Government Printing Office, 1987.
3. U.S. Bureau of the Census. Projections of the populations of the United States, by age, sex, and race, 1983 to 2080. *Current population reports*. Series P-25, No 952. Washington, DC: US Government Printing Office, 1984.
4. Torrey BB, Kinsella K, Taeuber CM. An aging world. *International population reports*. Series P-95, No 78. Washington, DC: US Government Printing Office, 1987.
5. National Center for Health Statistics. Advance report of final mortality statistics, 1987. *Monthly vital statistics report*, Vol 38 No 5 Suppl. Hyattsville, MD: Public Health Service, 1989.
6. Rosenwaike J. *The extreme aged in America*. Westpoint, CT: Greenwood Press, 1985.
7. National Center for Health Statistics. Multiple causes of death in the United States. *Monthly vital statistics report*, Vol 32, No 10 Suppl (2). DHHS Publication No (PHS) 84-1120. Hyattsville, MD: Public Health Service, 1984.

8. United Nations. *Demographic yearbook, 1984.* Publication No ST/ESA/STA/SER.R/14. New York: United Nations, 1986.
9. National Center for Health Statistics, Graves EJ. Utilization of short-stay hospitals, United States, 1984, annual summary. *Vital and health statistics*, Series 13, No 84. DHHS Publication No (PHS) 86-1745. Washington, DC: US Government Printing Office, 1986.
10. Havlik RJ. Determinants of health—cardiovascular risk factors. In: reference 2, p 39.
11. National Center for Health Statistics and National Heart, Lung and Blood Institute Collaborative Lipid Group. Trends in serum cholesterol level among US adults aged 20 to 74 years. *JAMA* 1987;257:937–42.
12. National Center for Health Statistics, Collins JG. Prevalence of selected chronic conditions, United States, 1979–81. *Vital and health statistics*, Series 10, No 155. DHHS Publication No (PHS) 86-1583. Washington, DC: US Government Printing Office, 1986.
13. National Center for Health Statistics, Harris T. Aging in the eighties: prevalence and impact of urinary problems in individuals age 65 years and over. Preliminary data from the Supplement on Aging to the National Health Interview Survey, United States, January–June 1984. *Advance data from vital and health statistics*, No 121. DHHS Publication No (PHS) 86-1250. Hyattsville, MD: Public Health Service, 1986.
14. National Center for Health Statistics, Havlik RJ. Aging in the eighties: impaired senses for sound and light in persons age 65 years and over. Preliminary data from the Supplement on Aging to the National Health Interview Survey, United States, January–June 1984. *Advance data from vital and health statistics*, No 125. DHHS Publication No (PHS) 86-1250. Hyattsville, MD: Public Health Service, 1986.
15. National Center for Health Statistics, Fitte JE, Kovar MG. Supplement on aging, 1984 National Health Interview Survey. *Vital and health statistics*, Series 1, No 21. Hyattsville, MD: Public Health Service.
16. Wilson B, Kovar MG, Havlik RJ. Health status and determinants-marriage, living alone, and risk to institutionalization. In: reference 2, p 27.
17. National Center for Health Statistics, Hing E, Sekscenski E, Strahan G. The National Nursing Home Survey; 1985 summary for the United States. *Vital and health statistics*, Series 13, No 97. DHHS Publication No (PHS) 86-1758. Washington, DC: US Government Printing Office.
18. Kemper P, Murtaugh C. Lifetime use of nursing home care. *N Engl J Med* 1991;324:595–600.
19. Rowe JW, Kahn RL. Human aging: usual and successful. *Science* 1987;237:143–9.
20. Havlik RJ. Physical, social and mental vitality in older persons. In: Feinleib M, ed. Proceedings of 1988 International Symposium on Data on Aging, National Center for Health Statistics. *Vital Health Stat* 1991;5(6):215–22.
21. Radloff LS, Teri L. Use of the Center for Epidemiological Studies—depression scale with older adults. In: Brink TL, ed. *Clinical gerontology.* New York: The Haworth Press, 1986:119–36.
22. Fries JF, Crapo LM. *Vitality and aging.* San Francisco: Freeman, 1981.

DISCUSSION

Dr. Chandra: It is important to gain a better idea of the number of elderly persons in developing countries and by how much they are affected by disability. In a WHO workshop in India about 4 years ago it was stated that at least 4% of the Asian population is above 65 years of age; of these, one-third may have disabling problems.

Dr. Havlik: The WHO is active in this area and has set up a field station responsible for a specialized program on aging. There is particular interest in Alzheimer's disease, which is underreported, as well as osteoporosis and the concept of "healthy aging." A protocol is at present under review with the aim of developing objective measures of disability that are independent of culture. In our own local studies we have tried to derive performance measures to standardize such activities as the ability to get up from a sitting position and to walk back and forth in a particular time. There is a great need to identify how many old people are truly disabled by aging diseases; having done so, it will of course be possible to estimate the numbers of people who are aging reasonably well.

Dr. Chandra: There is also a need to improve the precision of diagnosis of causes of death. However, infection such as pneumonia is a frequent terminal event and the immediate cause of death; this is usually not recorded. It is possible that progressive changes in the immune system may result in increased susceptibility to infection. This could be a common factor in many terminal illnesses.

Dr. Havlik: The issue of multiple causes of death is indeed a problem, and it may be very difficult to establish the pathogenesis of terminal illnesses in old age. In the United States there is a particular problem in nursing homes, where the attending physician often has no idea what the cause of death is, and so tends to put down "heart failure" or some other generalization. This is not really acceptable but is a practical reality. We are trying to improve the situation by increasing the autopsy rate in old people and by trying to make geriatricians aware of the significance of what they enter on death certificates.

Dr. Guesry: In the USA you have the advantage of having a multicultural, multiracial community. Do you find differences in the importance attached to the social and family role of the elderly in the various different sections of the community? In certain cultures, for example, elderly people have a more important role in the family and in raising young children than in others. They are, thus, socially more important and I wonder whether this plays a role in their survival.

Dr. Havlik: This is an important issue and there is a large behavioral and social research program in our institute examining such factors. There is no doubt that married men tend to live longer than those who are divorced or single, although this may reflect factors concerned with those who do not marry. The Hispanic community in the USA has traditionally been a stronger family than the other ethnic groups, but whether there is a difference between, for example, Mexican Americans as compared to Mexicans is not clear. In the current national survey we are sampling Hispanics, blacks, and whites so that we shall be able to compare health and family histories in these three groups.

Dr. Steen: We have for over two decades performed longitudinal studies in the elderly and have found no indication that a high body weight or high total cholesterol is a risk factor for mortality from age 70 years onward. I am unhappy about the American and Australian way of thinking in relation to these factors—measuring total cholesterol says nothing in mortality terms for a 70-year-old woman, who is the most likely person to go and have her cholesterol taken. Have you any firm data that cholesterol is a risk factor beyond the age of 70?

Dr. Havlik: As far as cholesterol is concerned, I agree that it is a challenge of the cholesterol education program to clarify this issue. As more cases have accumulated in the older age group, it appears that total cholesterol is still a predictor in the 60s, but more information on the fractionated lipoprotein pattern is needed. So far as weight is concerned, if Dr. Reubin Andres from our Gerontology Research Center was here he would have emphasized again the issue of the U-shaped curve, with optimal weight increasing in later life, and the importance of not using young adults as a standard. However, we do not yet have enough data on the over 70s from our national surveys to be sure about the predictive value of overweight in this age group.

Dr. Nestel: I disagree with Dr. Steen about the significance of hypercholesterolemia in the elderly. There is considerable evidence (1–3) that the risk in men, and to a lesser extent women, over the age of 65 is as great as for middled-aged people. In Australia the decline in mortality between the mid-1960s and the mid-1980s was 50% for elderly men and women, exactly the same reduction as for middle-aged men and women. Thus, whatever has been responsible for reducing coronary heart disease mortality in younger people has also been reflected in older people.

Dr. Havlik: Nevertheless, Dr. Steen may still be saying that the data are not nearly so clear in old age and there may be more appropriate ways of maintaining health than a dramatic change of diet at this time of life.

Dr. Rush: Willett and colleagues have commented on the issue of body weight and survival in an article in the *American Journal of Clinical Nutrition* (4). He argues that the optimal weight/survival relationship may increase with age because the relationship is not adjusted for smoking. While smoking could account for the U-shape of the distribution of weight and survival, I see no reason why smoking could account for the rise in optimal weight with age.

Dr. Caballero: A survey published by Tayback *et al.* (5) showed that over the age of 65 mortality in overweight individuals was no different from that in normal-weight persons. Underweight was a higher risk factor than overweight. We should not disregard or minimize the risk of undernutrition in this age group in determining mortality.

REFERENCES

1. Benfante R, Reed D. Is elevated serum cholesterol level a risk factor for coronary heart disease in the elderly? *JAMA* 1990;263:393–6.
2. Castelli WP, Wilson PW, Levy D, Anderson K. Cardiovascular risk factors in the elderly. *Am J Cardiol* 1989;63:124–94.
3. Gordon DJ, Rifkind BM. Treating high blood cholesterol in the older patient. *Am J Cardiol* 1989;63: 484–524.
4. Willett WC, Stampfer M, Manson JA, Van Itallie T. New weight guidelines for Americans: justified or injudicious? *Am J Clin Nutr* 1991;53:1102–3.
5. Tayback M, Kumanyika S, Chee E. Body weight as a risk factor in the elderly. *Arch Intern Med* 1990;150:1065–72.

Nutrition of the Elderly, edited by H. Munro, and
G. Schlierf, Nestlé Nutrition Workshop Series, Vol. 29,
Nestec Ltd., Vevey/Raven Press, Ltd., New York © 1992.

Research on Food Habits and Aging in Different Cultures in Europe: An Exploration[1]

Wija A. van Staveren, Lisette (C). P.G.M. de Groot, and
Joseph G.A.J. Hautvast

*Department of Human Nutrition, Wageningen Agricultural University,
6700 EV Wageningen, The Netherlands*

The ultimate goal of research on "better nutrition and aging" is to improve quality of life for the elderly. Quality of life is a personal matter and depends on the various ways in which people live in different cultures, climates, and under different socio-economic conditions. Quality of life, however, as far as food and nutrition in the elderly are concerned, also means improving or maintaining health with good nutrition and enjoyable meals. Studies on dietary habits of older populations in various cultures and their health status may provide insight in which factors might be involved in the relation between nutrition and quality of life in the elderly.

The European community (EC) concerted action on nutrition and health initiated a study in elderly people in Europe on food habits, aspects of lifestyle, and health because of the great variety of existing food patterns, environmental factors, and medical characteristics in people in different European countries and sometimes also within these countries (1). This chapter concentrates on problems we encountered in assessing cross-cultural food habits—the selection of a method, the development of a questionnaire, treatment of data, including conversion into energy and nutrients, and what these problems mean for the interpretation of some results.

OBJECTIVE AND DESIGN OF THE EUROPEAN STUDY

The European study on nutrition and the elderly was defined as "an explorative study on dietary patterns in the elderly living in different European communities, in relation to health and performance." Regarding food habits, the research questions were:

---

[1] The work discussed in this chapter is part of the Euronut SENECA Study on Nutrition and Health of the Elderly in Europe.

What are the differences in food habits (purchases, preparation, meal patterns, food avoidances, and supplement use) in the different communities studied?

What is the extent of differences in intake of energy, nutrients, and foods of elderly people living in these communities?

Nineteen centers in 12 countries agreed to participate (see the map in Fig. 1). The centers were asked to select a "traditional" small town with 10,000 to 20,000 inhabitants. By "traditional" was meant one with limited immigration. Moreover, the selected town should have a socioeconomic structure comparable to that in the country as a whole. The design of the study allowed for partial participation of two birth-year cohorts (1913, 1914) and complete participation involving six birth-year cohorts (1913–1918). The latter design was planned in order to conduct a follow-up study. The number of subjects aimed for, 60 in the partial study and 220 in the complete study, was selected randomly from the eligible population by a standardized procedure. For a complete description of the design of the study see reference 2.

Selection of the Method and Design of the Questionnaire

The aim of the European study in the elderly required information on food consumption, energy intake, and nutrient intake to be related to data on the nutritional status and health as well as on habits in food purchases, preparation, food avoidances, use of therapeutic diets, and any other food habits that might be relevant to adequate or inadequate nutrition.

An adapted dietary history method was selected to assess meal patterns, food patterns, and energy and nutrient intake. It is well known that a dietary history gives information on the habitual food intake rather than the actual food intake. For this study this was the required piece of information, but the disadvantage of this method is that the quality of the data collected depends on the capacity of the individuals to recall their habitual food pattern (3). Some principle investigators in the study doubted if it would be possible to collect valid data by this method. Therefore, we decided to combine the method with a 3-day record method. The elderly participants were asked to complete these records before the dietary history interview. This combination of methods had the advantage that participants had thought about their food consumption and were less likely to forget important foods during the interview. Furthermore, the interviewer could use the 3-day record for questions on the dietary patterns and food use. The reference time in the dietary history was the past month, portion sizes of foods frequently used were checked by weighing, and conversion into nutrients was done by using local food tables. The method was validated against a 3-day weighed method. Food habits were assessed by a general questionnaire. About 20 questions on shopping, meal preparation, visits to restaurants, use of (prescribed) diet, avoidance of special foods, use of health foods, drinking habits, and so on were incorporated in the general questionnaire.

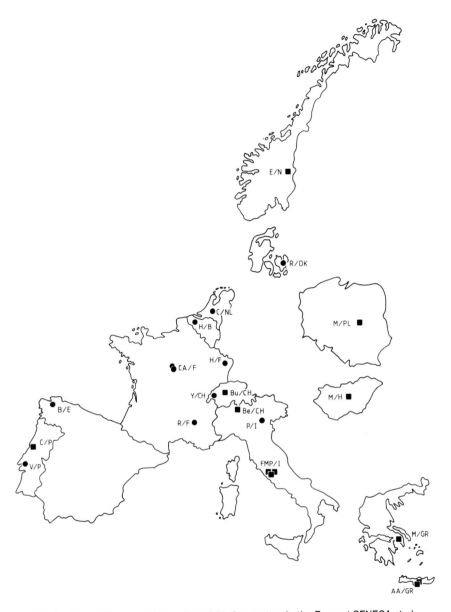

FIG. 1. Map of Europe with the 19 participating centers in the Euronut-SENECA study.

Standardization of the Method

Much attention has been paid to standardization of the questionnaires used in this study. A working group developed and worked out the adapted dietary history and questionnaire on food habits in English. The questionnaires were translated into the local language, after which they were tried out in the field by all participating centers and returned with comments to the coordinating center. A training course was then organized in which the persons responsible for the field work in all the centers participated. The aim of the course was to reach agreement and understanding of all the questions used. As a final check all the questionnaires were translated back into English.

Problems Encountered in the Treatment and Interpretation of Data

The dietary history should give information on meal patterns and mean daily food, energy, and nutrient intakes.

Meal Patterns

The problem with assessing meal patterns was that not all centers were able to work with meal codes. For these centers we have data on only mean food and nutrient intake per day. Nevertheless, for detecting characteristic differences between meal patterns in Europe, a sufficient number of centers have been able to use a meal code. For instance, in three centers most subjects eat on three occasions during the day and some subjects eat only twice. This is in contrast with two other centers—in more well-to-do countries—in which the majority of elderly people eat five or six times during the day and sometimes as often as eight times. This leads to large differences of energy intakes per meal. In the near future we may test one or more hypotheses on the effect of nibbling versus meal eating on these subjects (4).

Foods

For describing foods used during the day and at meal times we used the Eurocode (5), which can be attached to all European nutrient databases. However, for the

---

FIG. 2. Mean intake of calcium **(A)**, milk and milk products (butter and cheese not included) **(B)**, and cheese **(C)** in elderly people aged 70 to 75 years living in 14 of the 19 participating centers in the Euronut-SENECA study. Abbreviations: B, Hamme, Belgium; DK, Roskilde, Denmark; FS, Hagenau, Strasbourg, France; GrA, Markopoulo, Greece, near Athens; GrI, Anogio, Archanes Iraklion-Crete; H, Monor, Hungary; I, Italy, near Rome; N1, Culemborg, Netherlands; N, Elverum, Norway; P, Villa Franca de Xira Portugal; E, Bestanzos, Spain; CHY, Yverdon, Switzerland; GHBu, Burgdorf, Switzerland; CHBe, Bellinzona, Switzerland.

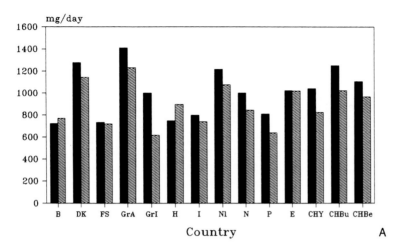

A

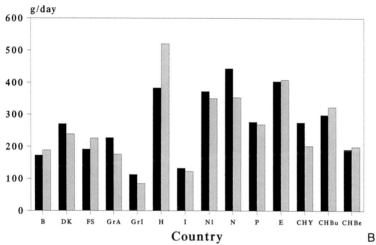

B

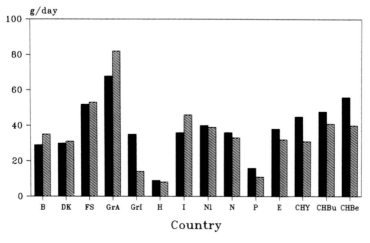

■ men ▨ women

C

description of foods we could only use the main food groups: milk, eggs, meat, poultry, fish, fats and oils, grains, vegetables and fruits, pulses and seeds, sugar and sugar products, beverages, alcoholic drinks, and food for special nutritional use (diet products). This information gives us a rough idea of the main sources of nutrients. Only major differences between centers could be detected; for instance, differences in calcium intake as determined by intake of dairy products (see Fig. 2A–C, preliminary data). Difficulties encountered in this field are, among others: (i) inconsistencies in the Eurocode that made it impossible to include all foods used and reported in the study, and (ii) the categorization of mixed dishes in raw ingredients taking into account nutrient losses and gains during food preparation.

Nutrient Databases

It was decided to use local nutrient databases for the conversion of foods into nutrients, because of the expected differences in the different national food composition tables, especially with regard to manufactured foods. It was recognized that there are many inconsistencies between these tables due either to different systems of analysis or sampling procedures, or to differences in factors applied to convert analyzed values to nutrients. Since it was important to know how nutrients were calculated in the different centers, a short questionnaire was developed to investigate the differences that exist between the food composition tables in the various centers. The differences considered were:

- the conversion of macronutrients into energy
- the conversion factors for nitrogen into protein
- the determination of carbohydrates, and data available on polysaccharides and mono- and disaccharides
- the determination of dietary fiber
- the nature of the fatty acids included in saturated, monounsaturated, and polyunsaturated fatty acids and the way in which fatty acids are expressed (e.g., in g fat/100 g fat or in g fatty acids/100 g fat)
- the use of retinol equivalents.

The effects of differences in food composition tables were checked using a sample of the food intake data from three countries. The data from Hungary, Norway, and Portugal were converted into energy and macronutrients by the local database as well as by the Dutch nutrient composition database. The test was conducted only with macronutrients because it was hypothesized that true or biological differences between foods would mainly exist among the micronutrients. Table 1 shows the differences found with this procedure. The differences were all less than 10% for the components considered. This was not as great as we had expected.

TABLE 1. *Difference in means of energy and macronutrient intakes of 21 elderly people from three centers in Europe, as calculated using the Dutch nutrient database and local nutrient databases*

Food components		Local data minus Dutch data		Difference %[a]
		Mean	90% confidence limits	
Energy	MJ	0.6	0.4; 0.9	9
Protein	g	4.4	1.8; 7.1	7
Fatty acids				
Saturated	g	0.4	−2.2; 3.6	2
Monounsaturated	g	0.02	−2.6; 2.6	0
Polyunsaturated	g	−0.2	−1.2; 0.9	−2
Carbohydrates	g	17.1	7.7; 26.6	8
Dietary fiber	g	−0.8	−2.8; 1.3	−5

[a] Difference as percentage of the local nutrient database.

Questionnaire on Food Habits

The main problems in assessing food habits in this European study were differences in the translation and interpretation of the questions. The list in Table 2 shows the most common translation problems, which were detected by translating the local questionnaire back into English. From this list it is clear that some problems are more serious than others (e.g., animal products may actually be the expensive foods). The fact that errors appear in different parts of the questionnaire must generate caution in the interpretation of the results. In addition to mistakes in the translation, errors of interpretation may also exist and may be caused by the fact that some items have alternative meanings in the various cultures. Some examples of possible pitfalls are discussed below.

Example 1. According to the question on food purchases, more than 75% of the subjects had shopping facilities close by or within walking distance. Shopping prob-

TABLE 2. *Examples of translation errors in the questionnaire used in the Euronut-SENECA study*

Description of items	English questionnaire	Local questionnaire
Foods	Canned foods	Tinned foods
	Expensive products	Animal products
	Health food	Natural foods
Meat	Burned meat	Grilled, roasted, or browned
Margarines	Diet margarine or high in PUFA	Low fat
Dairy	Buttermilk	Dairy cream, whey
Plant products	Fruit	Greens
Supplements	Doses in micrograms	Doses in 10^{-1} micrograms
Dentures	Removable	Natural

lems were more often due to budgeting problems than to the availability of shops. The fact that distance to shops was not a major problem for food shopping may reflect the selection of a "traditional town" by the study design. It is clear that budgeting problems may cause difficulties in shopping. It is not clear, however, how serious the problem is in our study, because the item "shopping" has been translated erroneously in a few centers (translated as a question on the availability of money rather than the availability of shops, which was the original question).

Example 2. Also connected with the use of "traditional towns" in the study design might be the fact that in all but one center half or more of the elderly participants consumed home-produced foods. Some preliminary data suggest that the use of home-produced foods is advantageous for dietary intakes as well as for health status (6). Whether "the use of home-produced foods" means production by elderly people themselves or mainly by family or friends needs to be examined. Furthermore, it is important to determine whether the apparent positive consequences for health status are related to physical activity or to dietary intakes or both.

Example 3. For the great majority of elderly people in all centers, the preferred place of eating is their own home. Interest in food preparation and in a daily cooked meal is sometimes used as a quick indicator for an inadequate diet (7). Problems may arise in cross-cultural comparisons due to the fact that in some cultures two cooked meals per day are traditional whereas in others only one cooked meal per day will be consumed. For instance, in the Netherlands only one cooked meal per day is eaten and, moreover, it is regular practice that on Saturday no cooked meals are consumed at all. (The kitchen should be kept clean for Sunday.) If we want to test in this study the hypothesis that irregular meal patterns are related to inadequate dietary intakes, then the term "irregular meal pattern" should be defined differently for the various centers.

CONCLUSION

In this chapter we have discussed some of the problems in assessing food habits cross-culturally. The chapter is based on problems of this kind encountered in the European study on nutrition and health in the elderly. Among these were the following:

- problems with the standardization of the dietary history
- problems with compatibility between the national food composition tables
- problems with the translation of the questionnaire into the local language and the adaptation according to local practice
- problems with the interpretation of the results in the various cultures.

ACKNOWLEDGMENT

We are greatly indebted to Dr. Haller from Hoffmann-La Roche & Co Ltd. for the translation of the local questionnaires back into English. We would also like to thank Desiree Welten for her help in the comparison of nutrient data bases of the various centers.

REFERENCES

1. Heikkinen E, Waters WE, Brezinski ZJ. The elderly in eleven countries: a sociomedical survey. Public Health Reports No 21. Copenhagen: WHO, 1987.
2. Groot CPGM de, Staveren WA van. Nutrition and the elderly: manual of operations for a European collaborative study. Wageningen: EURONUT Report No 11, 1988.
3. Cameron ME, Staveren WA van. *Manual on methodology for food consumption studies.* Oxford: Oxford University Press, 1988.
4. Jenkins DJA, Wolever TMS, Vuksan V, *et al.* Nibbling versus gorging: metabolic advantages of increased meal frequency. *N Engl J Med* 1989;321:929–34.
5. Arab L, Wittler M, Schettler G. *European food composition tables in translation.* Berlin: Springer–Verlag, 1987.
6. Schlettwein-Gsell D, Dirren H, Decarli B, *et al.* Ernährung und Ernährungsstatus von 361 70–75 jährigen Betagten in drei Regionen der Schweiz. in 3. Schweiz. Ernährungsbericht III, 225–79.
7. Davies L. Risk factors for malnutrition. In: Horwitz A, MacFadyen DM, Steen B, Williams TF, eds. *Nutrition in the elderly.* Oxford: Oxford University Press, 1989:153–66.

DISCUSSION

Dr. Steen: Your study is a major contribution to the understanding of transcultural food habits. Could you say something about how representative your results were? What information do you have about non-response?

Dr. van Staveren: This is an important question. Response was certainly a problem in some centers. We had centers with 100% response and others with only 50%. We did a small non-response survey that indicated that health and education were factors in non-response. Our statistician adjusted for these factors but we did not find large differences between the weighted medians and the "raw" (or "unweighted") data for many of the questions posed.

Dr. Hodkinson: Why did you choose small towns of 10,000 to 20,000? It seems to me that in industrialized countries such small towns are likely to be rather non-representative of the general population.

Dr. van Staveren: We expected that if we examined the smaller traditional towns we would find greater differences in dietary patterns.

Dr. Berry: I think this is a remarkable study but it does highlight the problems of finding objective markers of dietary intake. Will you have an opportunity to proceed with some "invasive" procedures? By this I mean blood testing for albumin, transport proteins, and maybe T_3 concentrations, and possibly adipose tissue biopsy for fatty acid analysis for the quality of dietary fat? This is a relatively non-invasive procedure, it does not hurt, and it has the advantage over blood testing that you can never miss!

Dr. van Staveren: We are well acquainted with the use of fat biopsies, but we did not do them in this study. However, we have blood samples and intend to validate some of the dietary findings against them, although we have not done this yet.

Dr. Guesry: The countries in your survey come from an area stretching almost from the North Pole down to the south of Greece. I assume there are huge differences in diet in these different countries. It is commonly said that the Mediterranean diet is healthier than other diets, but I wonder if this is because the circumstances of life have changed less in the

Mediterranean than they have in northern Europe. In other words, could it be that the diet is no longer well adapted to lifestyle in the industrialized parts of Europe, and that it is more difficult to change diet than it is to change lifestyle?

Dr. van Staveren: Our study will not answer this question but I believe that there are other studies that show that diets rich in saturated fats are compatible with good health in people doing heavy physical work.

Dr. Meredith: How did you deal with the problem of reliability of reporting in older people with impaired memory? And was there a seasonal influence on your results?

Dr. van Staveren: People with dementia were not involved, and the study was done in only one season, the winter.

Dr. Steen: It is appropriate to mention that a transcultural study of nutrition in the elderly is at present underway under the auspices of the International Union of Nutritional Sciences. Studies of eating behavior are taking place in several countries, for example China, Greece, Australia, Sweden, Iceland, and some African countries, and in communities in the vicinity of New York and in Texas. One of the purposes of this transcultural study is not only to measure nutrient intakes, but also to assess the ways in which food is eaten—with whom, where, in what surroundings, and so on.

Dr. Nestel: Have you distinguished between n-6 and n-3 fatty acids? There is a tendency to lump them together but we now know it is very important to distinguish between them, in the light of recent studies showing an inverse correlation between n-3 fatty acid intake and mortality from a variety of diseases, including coronary artery disease and some cancers.

Dr. van Staveren: This will have to be the subject of a special project due to the problems I have already shown relating to local food composition tables. However, we are very interested in this subject and plan to investigate it, if not in all centers then at least in some of them.

Dr. Havlik: In terms of future studies, are there any plans to do substudies in certain centers and is the European Community working to produce a common set of food tables that can be used throughout Europe?

Dr. van Staveren: Subsidiary studies will certainly be done in several centers. For example, some will perform a more extensive evaluation of hematology, others of bone density, immunology, and so on.

As to food tables, the European community is supporting a project to make these more compatible between EC countries. We are at present working hard on this.

Dr. Schlierf: When evaluating data on energy intake it is important to know something about energy expenditure. How did you do this?

Dr. van Staveren: We administered a questionnaire on physical activity that we validated against other measures. We were not able to quantify energy expenditure but there were some interesting differences between centers in time spent on various activities.

Dr. Edwardson: Did you collect any data on past eating habits? Historically, the patterns of eating are changing quite dramatically even in quite small communities and if the health of old people is in some way dependent on their lifetime nutritional experience, then maybe the variation over, say, the last 40 years is more important than the current cultural variation.

Dr. Davies: This is one of the questions that has been taken up in the IUNS studies mentioned by Dr. Steen. We are examining past as well as present food habits and food beliefs.

Dr. Steen: The question of beliefs about food is a very important one and is one of the most prominent differences between countries. In a rather sterile country like my own, people do not tend to have many beliefs about what is good or bad to eat, but in countries like Greece or China there are hundreds of food items that are believed to be good or bad for your health. This is one of the major differences between countries.

Dr. van Staveren: It is clear from our data that it is more common for people to avoid foods for health than it is for them to eat foods for health.

Nutrition of the Elderly, edited by H. Munro, and
G. Schlierf, Nestlé Nutrition Workshop Series, Vol. 29,
Nestec Ltd., Vevey/Raven Press, Ltd., New York © 1992.

Renal Function and Histopathology in the Elderly

Hiroshi Sato, Takao Saito, and Kaoru Yoshinaga

The Second Department of Internal Medicine, Tohoku University School of Medicine, Sendai City, 980, Miyagi, Japan

AGING AND RENAL FUNCTION

Decline of renal function with aging is the most dramatic among all the organ systems. Functioning cells are gradually lost and physiologic reserve capacity is reduced. The glomerular filtration rate, which is low at birth, approaches adult level by 3 years, and is maintained at approximately 140 ml/min/1.73 m² until the age of 25 to 34 years. Thereafter, it declines linearly by approximately 8 ml/min/1.73 m² per decade (1,2). The glomerular filtration rate of healthy octagenarians is only half or two-thirds of that measured in young adults.

These functional changes are accompanied by corresponding structural changes in the kidney. The two kidneys, which weigh approximately 50 g at birth, increase to between 270 g and 350 g in the third and fourth decades, but subsequently decline to less than 200 g by the ninth decade. The loss of renal mass is principally initiated in the cortex, with relative sparing of the medulla.

The number of functioning glomeruli declines roughly in accord with the changes in renal weight. Up to the age of 40 years, sclerotic glomeruli constitute less than 5% of the total. With increasing age thereafter, the incidence of sclerotic glomeruli increases, so that sclerosis involves 10% to 40% of the total glomerular population by the eighth decade (3–5). Kasiske (6) has shown that the mean percentage of sclerotic glomeruli in 60-year-old subjects with minimal vascular disease was approximately 5%, and that the number of obsolete glomeruli correlates directly with the severity of atherosclerosis. However, the size of the remaining glomeruli with no sclerosis increases with age (7,8), and is associated with ultrastructural and biochemical alterations of the glomerular constituents (to be discussed later in this chapter).

The precise mechanisms of the age-related changes in the kidney have not hitherto been elucidated. At least two separate subcomponents seem to exist in the aging process of the kidney. One component is an essential renal change resulting from the natural aging process, and is common to all human beings to some degree. Another is the influence of some pathophysiological conditions that can take place

29

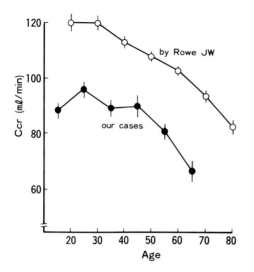

FIG. 1. Cross-sectional difference in creatinine (Ccr) clearance value with age. Values plotted indicate mean ± SEM. ○, mean value in each age group studied by Rowe *et al.* (1) on normal subjects (n = 548); ●, mean value in our study on patients with chronic glomerulonephritis (n = 215).

intermittently or continuously throughout the person's life. Hypertension, dehydration, drug abuse, glomerulonephritis due to immunologic injury, and various infections including pyelonephritis would be examples of such conditions (9,10). Lindeman (10) suggested that nephropathic environmental factors or common pathologic processes were mainly responsible for the age-related renal dysfunction. Virtually all the histological changes observed in the aged kidney may be induced not only by the natural aging process but also by miscellaneous pathologic factors such as those mentioned above. There is great difficulty in distinguishing the purely age-related effects from the other effects. It is thus inevitable that the ensuing discussion relates to renal changes in general without defining or analyzing specific etiologies.

Our study on patients with chronic glomerulonephritis has revealed an age-dependent decline in renal function, evaluated by creatinine clearance value (Fig. 1). The gradient of renal function decrease in our study is quite similar to that shown by Rowe *et al.* (1), who studied healthy adults without any specific renal diseases. From this observation, the aging process is assumed to have effects on all individuals whether or not they suffer from renal disease.

RENAL MORPHOLOGICAL CHANGES IN THE ELDERLY

Several investigators have shown that there is an increase in the mesangial matrix and a progressive thickening or folding of the glomerular basement membrane (GBM) and tubular basement membrane in the aged kidney (2,7,11–13). Figure 2 shows our results of ultrastructural examinations on the GBM thickness in 167 patients with renal diseases, excluding membranous glomerulonephritis, hereditary nephritis, diabetes, amyloidosis, and transplanted kidney. The method of Osawa *et al.* (14) was used in measuring GBM thickness. As shown in this figure, the GBM thickness

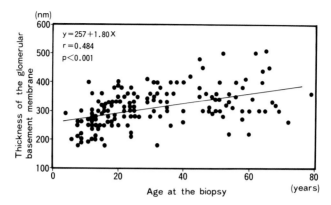

FIG. 2. Correlation between the thickness of the glomerular basement membrane (GBM) and the age at the time of biopsy (n = 167). The GBM thickness significantly increases with age.

increases with age. In Cockayne's syndrome (15), a congenital anomaly character-ized by the accelerated aging process of multiple organs, the GBM is extremely thickened to approximately 3 times the normal thickness. These intraglomerular mor-phological changes are probably associated with an age-related increase in extra-cellular material such as laminine and type IV collagen, which is the main component of the GBM and mesangial matrix (16,17). Furthermore, biochemical analysis of the GBM demonstrates decreased sulfation of the glycosaminoglycans, an alteration that could reduce the net negative charge and render the GBM more permeable to mac-romolecules (18), leading to an increase in urinary protein excretion and to a pro-gressive glomerular sclerosis (19,20).

The functional and morphological interglomerular imbalance that develops with aging is also an important factor in the progression of glomerular sclerosis. Thus, as sclerosis progresses, some glomeruli fall into capillary collapse or segmental scle-rosis, resulting in a decreased filtration rate, while the remaining glomeruli show morphological hypertrophy and functional hyperfiltration in an attempt to preserve the total kidney function. This compensatory hyperfiltration is assumed to be one of the main mechanisms of progressive glomerulosclerosis; it induces further GBM injury, cellular impairment, and an expansion of the mesangial matrix (2,21).

Figure 3 shows schematically the many paths leading to the development of glo-merular sclerosis. The aging process, as well as the presence of systemic hyperten-sion, diabetes, hyperlipidemia, arteriosclerosis, and so forth, is an important factor behind the multi-faceted incidence of glomerular injury. Furthermore, food intake is also a variable that can have considerable effects. In various experimental models that included aging animals of many species, the degree and the frequency of the glomerular sclerosis were affected by dietary manipulations. Limitation of total en-ergy intake was originally shown to delay the development of glomerular lesions (22,23). Afterward, a low protein diet (20–23) and restriction of dietary phosphorus (24) were shown to reduce proteinuria and to delay the age-related glomerular

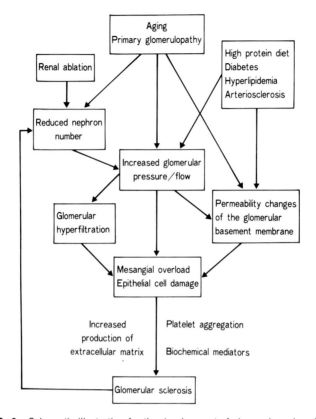

FIG. 3.   Schematic illustration for the development of glomerular sclerosis.

sclerosis, even when total energy intake was not restricted. It seems likely that dietary intake of carbohydrates in humans has little effect on the kidney, whereas protein intake influences renal size, structure, and function, mediated by intrarenal hemodynamic alterations (2,21). Renal blood flow and glomerular filtration rate rise with a high protein diet (25), resulting in renal hypertrophy. Brenner *et al.* (21) suggested that the protein-rich diet characteristic of modern Western society can alone induce chronic renal hyperfiltration and hyperperfusion and thereby contribute to the functional and structural deterioration of the aging kidney.

EVENTUAL RENAL FAILURE IN THE ELDERLY

In aged adults, not only glomerular filtration rate but also urine concentrating ability and the adaptive capacity for responding to changes in the intake of electrolytes and water are significantly impaired (26). Thus, various abnormal conditions such as overhydration, dehydration, or electrolyte imbalance are easily brought on by only a mild exogenous or endogenous stimulus, for example, bacterial or viral infection, surgical operation, decreased water intake, drug ingestion, and so forth (most of these events might be completely harmless to healthy young adults). In particular, a state of dehydration, which is easily and frequently induced without any subjective symptoms in older patients, may facilitate the expression of nephrotoxicity of various drugs, such as antibiotics, diuretics, contrast media, and non-steroidal anti-inflammatory drugs (NSAIDs), and can sometimes result in severe renal failure. Figure 4 shows the clinical course of a 64-year-old nephrotic patient who developed acute renal insufficiency after the combined administration of NSAIDs and diuretics. Creatinine clearance decreased from 57 to 13 ml/min, and blood pressure was significantly increased, probably due to water retention. The aged kidney is clearly at high risk of eventual failure, especially when the number of functioning nephrons is further reduced by acquired renal diseases.

Another problem is the discrepancy of the relationship between serum creatinine and the creatinine clearance value. The reduction in creatinine clearance with age is accompanied by a reduction in creatinine production, which reflects the decrease of muscle in body mass that occurs with age (1). Therefore, the relationship of serum creatinine to creatinine clearance changes with age; although creatinine clearance

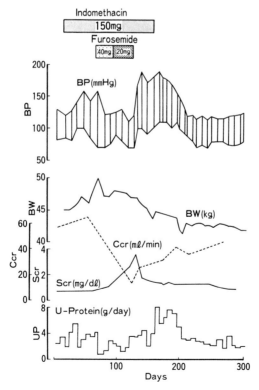

FIG. 4. Adverse effects of combined administration of indomethacin and furosemide on renal function, observed in a nephrotic 64-year-old woman with membranous glomerulonephritis.

decreases from 120 ml/min at age 20 years to 60 ml/min at age 80 years, serum creatinine concentration remains nearly constant at a level of approximately 1 mg/dl. The approximate creatinine clearance in adult men can be derived from the serum creatinine value with the following formula:

$$Ccr = \frac{(140 - age)[lean\ body\ weight\ (kg)]}{72 \times serum\ creatinine\ (mg/dl)}$$

In adult women, the clearance is approximated by multiplying the calculated value by 0.85 (2,27). The practical implication of these observations is that kidney function in older patients may sometimes be unexpectedly decreased, even if they have a normal serum creatinine value. Renal function reserve capacity may be even further decreased (25). Consequently, it is important for clinicians to pay attention to renal function at all times during the medical treatment of aged patients.

ACQUIRED KIDNEY DISEASES IN THE ELDERLY

Finally, we would like to comment on the spectrum and the character of the superimposed kidney disease in the elderly. The incidence of primary renal disease in elderly people may not be significantly greater than in younger adults. However, in contrast to younger age groups, crescentic glomerulonephritis, renal vasculitis including periarteritis nodosa, membranous glomerulonephritis, diabetic nephropathy, and renal amyloidosis are relatively more common in patients over 60 years of age (28–30). Most of these diseases are frequently resistant to steroid therapy or other medical treatment, and tend to progress slowly or rapidly to end-stage renal failure. On the other hand, steroid-sensitive minimal change disease is still observed in approximately 10% of cases of the nephrotic syndrome in the elderly (29,30). Some cases of the membranous glomerulonephritis, crescentic glomerulonephritis, and renal vasculitis may also respond to steroids or other drugs. Therefore, even in the elderly, histological diagnosis by renal biopsy is required to decide on an adequate treatment procedure, as long as the condition of the patient permits the execution of such a biopsy.

REFERENCES

1. Rowe JW, Andres R, Tobin JD, Norris AH, Shock NW. The effect of age on creatinine clearance in men: a cross-sectional longitudinal study. *J Gerontol* 1976;31:155–63.
2. Anderson S, Brenner BM. Effects of aging on the renal glomerulus. *Am J Med* 1986;80:435–42.
3. Kaplan C, Pasternack B, Shah H, Gallo G. Age-related incidence of sclerotic glomeruli in human kidneys. *Am J Pathol* 1975;80:227–34.
4. Kappel B, Olson S. Cortical interstitial tissues and sclerosed glomeruli in the normal human kidney, related to age and sex. A quantitative study. *Virchows Arch [A]* 1980;387:271–7.
5. Akiyama M, Sakaguchi H. Morphological study of renal changes with age. *Jpn J Nephrol* 1990;32:751–6.
6. Kasiske BL. Relationship between vascular disease and age-associated changes in the human kidney. *Kidney Int* 1987;31:1153–9.
7. McLachlan MSF. The ageing kidney. *Lancet* 1978;ii:143–6.
8. Goyal VK. Changes with age in the human kidney. *Exp Gerontol* 1982;17:321–31.

9. Anderson S. Decline of renal function with age; mechanisms, risk factors and therapeutic implications. In: Oreopoulos DG, ed. *Geriatric nephrology*. Dordrecht: Martinus Nijhoff, 1986:57–71.
10. Lindeman RD. Renal physiology and pathophysiology of aging. *Am J Kidney Dis* 1990;16:275–82.
11. Bloom PM, Hartmann JF, Vernier RL. An electron microscopic evaluation of the width of normal glomerular basement membrane in man at various ages (abstract). *Anat Rec* 1959;133:251.
12. Vracko R. Effects of aging and diabetes on basal lamina thickness of six cell types. In: Kefalides NA, ed. *Biology and chemistry of basement membranes*. New York: Academic Press, 1978:483–93.
13. Yoshikawa N, Uehara S, Yamada K, *et al*. Clinicopathological correlations of persistent asymptomatic proteinuria. *Nephron* 1980;25:127–33.
14. Osawa G, Kimmelstiel P, Seiling V. Thickness of the glomerular basement membranes. *Am J Clin Pathol* 1966;45:7–20.
15. Sato H, Saito T, Kurosawa K, Ootaka T, Furuyama T, Yoshinaga K. Renal lesions in Cockayne's syndrome. *Clin Nephrol* 1988;29:206–9.
16. Martinez-Hernandez A, Amenta PS. The basement membrane in pathology. *Lab Invest* 1983;48: 656–77.
17. Karttunen T, Risteli J, Autio-Harmainen H, Risteli L. Effect of age and diabetes on type IV collagen and laminine in human kidney cortex. *Kidney Int* 1986;30:586–91.
18. Cohen MP, Ku L. Age-related changes in sulfation of basement membrane glycosaminoglycans. *Exp Gerontol* 1983;18:447–50.
19. Remuzzi G, Bertani T. Is glomerulosclerosis a consequence of altered glomerular permeability to macromolecules? *Kidney Int* 1990;38:384–94.
20. Bertani T, Zoja C, Abbate M, Rossini M, Remuzzi G. Age-related nephropathy and proteinuria in rats with intact kidneys exposed to diets with different protein content. *Lab Invest* 1989;60:196–204.
21. Brenner BM, Meyer TW, Hostetter TH. Dietary protein intake and the progressive nature of kidney disease. *N Engl J Med* 1982;307:652–60.
22. Saxton JA, Kimball GC. Relation of nephrosis and other diseases of albino rats to age and to modifications of diet. *Arch Pathol* 1941;32:951–65.
23. Tucker SM, Mason RL, Beauchene RE. Influence of diet and feed restriction on kidney function of aging male rats. *J Gerontol* 1976;31:264–70.
24. Barsotti G, Morelli E, Giannonni A, Guiducci A, Lupetti S, Giovannetti S. Restricted phosphorus and nitrogen intake to slow the progression of chronic renal failure, a controlled trial. *Kidney Int* 1983;24(suppl 16):278–84.
25. Bosch JP, Saccaggi A, Lauer A, Ronco C, Belledonne M, Glabman S. Renal function reserve in humans: effect of protein intake on glomerular filtration rate. *Am J Med* 1983;75:943–50.
26. Lindeman RD, Goldman R. Anatomic and physiologic age changes in kidney. *Exp Gerontol* 1986;21:379–406.
27. Cockcroft DW, Gault MH. Prediction of creatinine clearance from serum creatinine. *Nephron* 1976;16:31–41.
28. Kingswood JC, Banks RA, Tribe CR, Owen-Jones J, Mackenzie JC. Renal biopsy in the elderly: clinicopathological correlations in 143 patients. *Clin Nephrol* 1984;22:183–7.
29. Zech P, Colon S, Pointet P, Deteix P, Labeeuw M, Leitienne P. The nephrotic syndrome in adults aged over 60. *Clin Nephrol* 1982;17:232–6.
30. Sato H, Saito T, Furuyama T, Yoshinaga K. Histologic studies on the nephrotic syndrome in the elderly. *Tohoku J Exp Med* 1987;153:259–64.

DISCUSSION

Dr. Hodkinson: I should like to make a comment on creatinine. You made the point that the relationship of serum creatinine to renal function changes with age because of the reduction in muscle mass in old people. This deserves special emphasis. In some of our elderly patients with chronic illness there is so much wasting that a normal serum creatinine may be found in the presence of frankly abnormal renal function. We did some work a few years ago (1) that showed that urea was a better predictor of renal function than creatinine in old age even when creatinine is adjusted for body weight, which is really only saying that adjustment for body weight is not very good. The geriatrician's experience is quite different from the usual nephrological opinion that urea is useless and creatinine is the gold standard.

Dr. Chandra: I have a comment relating to possible mechanisms of changes in renal function with age. There are animal models of autoimmune renal diseases, some of which are genetic, in which deterioration in renal function can be prevented by a low-energy, low-protein diet. My hypothesis is that in some aging individuals, autoimmune processes, which can be induced by viral infections, may be the reason for deterioration in renal function. Such autoimmune processes may be modified or arrested by a low-protein or low-energy intake.

Dr. Havlik: Although I realize that in many cross-sectional models there is not an important relationship between dietary protein intake and blood pressure, I wonder whether there is any new information on this. Could there be a correlation between dietary protein intake and blood pressure to the extent that quite minor increases in blood pressure over a long period might influence renal function?

Dr. Sato: Systemic hypertension does not correlate with dietary protein. It is much more dependent on dietary salt intake. However, high-protein diet may cause intrarenal, intraglomerular hypertension, mediated by mesangial hyperfunction and intrarenal vascular reaction. Intraglomerular hypertension over a long period might induce progressive glomerular sclerosis and renal dysfunction.

Dr. Durnin: It seems unlikely that there would be a relationship between dietary protein intake and hypertension or any sort of renal dysfunction. I don't think there is any evidence to show that individuals with widely varying protein intake have any differences in kidney function.

Dr. Nestel: There is evidence from studies in vegetarians and in animal models that the type of protein can influence the blood pressure. Diets rich in plant proteins appear to lead to substantially lower blood pressures than diets rich in animal proteins, in the absence of any systematic change in mineral intake.

Dr. Sato: In cases of healthy adults, influence of dietary protein on renal function may be negligible. It seems unlikely that dietary protein alone can induce renal damage by itself. But, it is possible that a high-protein diet may accelerate the renal damage caused by other pathological factors. In other words, a protein-rich diet could be harmful to the kidney that is already affected by acquired renal diseases, particularly when glomerular filtration rate is evidently decreased. I believe a few elderly people must have acquired kidney disease with insidious and subclinical renal insufficiency. A lot of experimental and clinical studies demonstrated beneficial effects of a low-protein diet on the progression of renal failure (2–5). On the other hand, restriction of dietary protein may cause a malnutritional condition. So, careful consideration is required for practical diet programming.

REFERENCES

1. Denham MJ, Hodkinson HM, Fisher M. Glomerular filtration rate in sick elderly inpatients. *Age Ageing* 1975;4:32–6.
2. Maschio G, Oldrizzi I, Lessitore N, *et al.* Effects of dietary protein and phosphorus restriction on the progression of early renal failure. *Kidney Int* 1982;22:371–6.
3. El-Nahas AM, Masters-Thomas A, Brady SA, *et al.* Selective effect of low protein diet in chronic renal diseases. *Br Med J* 1984;289:1337–41.
4. Oldrizzi I, Rugiu C, Valvo L, *et al.* Progression of renal failure in patients with renal disease of diverse etiology on protein-restricted diet. *Kidney Int* 1985;27:553–7.
5. Acchiardo SR, Moore IW, Cockrell S. Does low protein diet halt the progression of renal insufficiency? *Clin Nephrol* 1984;25:289–94.

Nutrition of the Elderly, edited by H. Munro, and
G. Schlierf, Nestlé Nutrition Workshop Series, Vol. 29,
Nestec Ltd., Vevey/Raven Press, Ltd., New York © 1992.

Endocrine Function in the Elderly

H. Malcolm Hodkinson

University College London, London NWI OPE, England, United Kingdom

Many different changes in endocrine function with age have been described. To give just some of many possible examples, there are increases in the levels of growth hormone in women, rises in thyroid stimulating hormone, modest decreases in triiodothyronine, and increased sensitivity of response to antidiuretic hormone (1). Levels of norepinephrine rise (2) and there are altered circadian patterns for cortisol, norepinephrine, and growth hormone (3). There are falls in renin and aldosterone levels (4) and a rise in parathyroid hormone levels, although this seems to be entirely due to decreased renal excretion (5). Pancreatic polypeptide and gastrin show rises with age, although other gut hormones do not appear to change (6).

However, these and many other described changes are generally small and of doubtful importance in a practical sense. They are certainly dwarfed by the important and major changes in sex hormones and gonadotropins, and this chapter will therefore concentrate on this area.

Changes in sex hormones and trophic hormones occur in both sexes with aging. Obviously the changes are far more dramatic in women in relation to the abrupt cessation of estrogen secretion by the ovary at the time of menopause. However, although there is no abrupt change in testicular function with age, there is a gradual diminution of Leydig cell function so that testosterone levels fall progressively. Gonadotropins rise in both sexes in response to these falls in sex hormone production.

ESTROGENS IN POSTMENOPAUSAL WOMEN

Within a few months of menopause, levels of the most potent estrogen, estradiol, fall markedly, whereas those of estrone fall only a little so that it then becomes the main estrogen (7). The ovary loses its ability to convert androstenedione to estrone and testosterone to estradiol. The greatly reduced production of estradiol now relies on peripheral conversion of its plasma precursors estrone, androstenedione, and, to a smaller extent, testosterone, as there is no direct secretion by the ovaries or adrenals (8). Similarly, the production of estrone is almost entirely by peripheral conversion of circulating androstenedione in adipose tissue. Androstenedione is in turn secreted mainly by the adrenals, although ovarian secretion does continue at about half its premenopausal level (8). As adipocytes are the site of these peripheral conversions, estrogen production, particularly that of the more potent estradiol, is more efficient in obese postmenopausal women (9). This explains the protective effect of obesity against postmenopausal osteoporosis that has been shown in many studies.

ANDROGENS IN POSTMENOPAUSAL WOMEN

The postmenopausal ovary continues to produce the androgens androstenedione and testosterone, although at somewhat reduced rates (8), while adrenal secretion of these two hormones and of dihydroepiandrosterone continues unchanged (10). As conversion of androgens to estrogens in the ovary no longer takes place, the net result is that total androgen levels are somewhat higher.

GONADOTROPINS AFTER MENOPAUSE

Levels of luteinizing hormone (LH) and of follicle-stimulating hormone (FSH) reach a maximum some 2 to 3 years after menopause (7) and remain elevated through-out later life by approximately four- and sixfold, respectively (11). Administration of estrogens to postmenopausal women causes LH and FSH to fall, indicating that the feedback loop is still intact and that the elevations can be regarded as secondary to the changes in the sex steroid hormones (11).

SEX HORMONE AND GONADOTROPIN CHANGES IN MEN

Although there are no abrupt changes in men comparable to menopause in women, androgens do fall somewhat with age (12) so that the main androgen, testosterone, as well as α-dihydrotestosterone have lower blood levels in elderly men. There do not seem to be any corresponding changes in estrogen levels; estrone, the most important estrogen in men, shows no age relationship (13). The position regarding gonadotropins is less clear-cut, with some workers finding no change with age, whereas others report some increase in LH beyond the age of 60 years (13).

CONSEQUENCES OF MENOPAUSE

The physical consequences of menopause such as atrophic changes in the genital tract, breast, skin, and other organs and tissues influenced by estrogens are well recognized. No less important, however, are the many metabolic consequences of estrogen withdrawal, not all of which are so well appreciated. Osteoporosis is per-haps the most serious and obvious of such changes, but there are various other changes that we should examine.

Biochemical Changes Following Menopause

Many biochemical analyses show age changes that could confound or obscure changes due to menopause itself. However, studies of women in the age groups during which natural menopause is experienced allow us to compare age-matched groups of women who are premenopausal or postmenopausal and so to allow fully for age effect. McPherson and colleagues were among the first to look systematically for such menopausal effects (14). They found that 7 of the 17 analyses they studied showed significant changes attributable to menopause itself!

Links to Bone Metabolism

McPherson *et al.* found a group of changes that can be linked to postmenopausal osteoporosis. Serum alkaline phosphatase and calcium showed significant elevations and there was also a nonsignificant rise in serum inorganic phosphate. Similarly, Crilly and colleagues (15) found a significant rise in both serum alkaline phosphatase and the urinary excretion of hydroxyproline. Taken together, these findings point strongly to linkage to the phase of rapid postmenopausal bone loss consequent upon estrogen withdrawal and preventable by estrogen administration. Thus, extra calcium and phosphate are released from bone into the bloodstream by the increased osteoclastic activity. This also gives increased collagen removal by destruction of bone matrix, leading to increased excretion of its degradation product, hydroxyproline. As osteoblastic activity is highly geared to osteoclastic activity, the rise in alkaline phosphatase is also readily explicable. It is of interest that the rises in phosphate and calcium persist into old age, where women have significantly higher values than men (16).

Estrogen also appears to have other effects that are relevant to bone physiology. Osteomalacia is widely recognized as being far more likely to affect old women rather than men. This may be due to differences in vitamin D metabolism between the sexes, for elderly women have significantly lower values of serum 25-hydroxycholecalciferol than men even when differences in age, dietary intake of vitamin D, and sunlight exposure are fully allowed for (17). Furthermore, the difference is quite substantial: women have values about 70% of those of men when other factors are balanced.

Urea and Electrolytes

McPherson and his colleagues also found significant elevations of blood urea and of serum bicarbonate and sodium after menopause. The changes reduced the differences between men and women in each case, although significant but small sex differences remained. This would suggest that sex hormones have important influences on renal function.

They also found that serum iron and serum aspartate aminotransferase rose significantly postmenopausally, again having the effect of bringing values closer to those for men. The change in serum iron could perhaps be ascribed to the cessation of menstrual iron loss, but there is no obvious explanation for the change in aspartate aminotransferase.

Uric Acid

Others have shown a significant postmenopausal elevation of serum uric acid (18), confirming the nonspecific trend found by McPherson and colleagues (14). Again, this brings female values closer to those for males and is paralleled by a rising incidence of acute gout in older women.

CONCLUSION

By far the most impressive hormonal changes occurring with aging are the changes in sex hormones and gonadotropins after menopause. Reduced estrogens in older women set in motion many physiological changes, some of which appear to be seriously deleterious (most particularly those underlying the development of postmenopausal osteoporosis, which is perhaps better regarded as an integral part of normal aging than as a disease).

Other hormonal changes appear to be relatively minor in nature in comparison with these and, although they may be of academic interest, do not seem to have major practical importance.

REFERENCES

1. Randall JU, Veldhuis JD. Hypothalamo-pituitary concomitants of aging. In: Sowers JR, Felicetta JV, eds. *Endocrinology of aging.* New York: Raven Press, 1988:41–74.
2. Ziegler MG, Lake CR, Kopin IJ. Plasma noradrenalin increases with age. *Nature* 1976;261:333–5.
3. McGinty D, Stern N, Akshoomoff N. Circadian and sleep-related modulation of hormone levels. In: Sowers JR, Felicetta JV, eds. *Endocrinology of aging.* New York: Raven Press, 1988:75–111.
4. Hegstad R, Brown RD, Jiang N-S, *et al.* Aging and aldosterone. *Am J Med* 1983;74:442–8.
5. Marcus R, Madvig P, Young G. Age-related changes in parathormone and parathormone hormone actions in normal humans. *J Clin Endocrinol Metab* 1984;58:223–30.
6. Adrian T, Bloom SR. Gut and pancreatic hormones in the elderly. In: Hodkinson HM, ed. *Clinical biochemistry of the elderly.* Edinburgh: Churchill Livingstone, 1984:237–45.
7. Studd JWW, Chakravarti S, Collins WP. Plasma hormone profiles after the menopause and bilateral oophorectomy. *Postgrad Med J* 1978;(suppl 2):25–30.
8. Grodin JM, Siiteri PK, MacDonald PC. Source of oestrogen production in postmenopausal women. *J Clin Endocrinol Metab* 1973;36:207–14.
9. Jensen J, Riis BJ, Hummer L, Christiansen C. The effects of age and body composition on circulating serum oestrogens and androstenedione after the menopause. *Br J Obstet Gynaecol* 1985;92:260–5.
10. Mills T, Mahesh VB. Pituitary function in the aged. In: Greenblatt RB, ed. *Geriatric endocrinology,* Vol 5. New York: Raven Press, 1978:1–11.
11. Chakravarti S, Oram DH, Forecast J, Studd J. A study of gonadotropins after the menopause. *Br J Obstet Gynaecol* 1976;83:587–8.
12. Zumoff B, Strain GW, Kream J, *et al.* Age variation of the 24-hr mean plasma concentrations of

androgens, estrogens and gonadotropins in normal adult men. *J Clin Endocrinol Metab* 1982;54: 534–8.
13. Davidson JM, Chen JJ, Crapo L, Gray GD, Greenleaf WJ, Catania JA. Hormonal changes and sexual function in aging men. *J Clin Endocrinol Metab* 1983;57:71–7.
14. McPherson K, Healy MJR, Flynn FV, Piper KAJ, Garcia-Webb P. The effect of age, sex and other factors on blood chemistry in health. *Clin Chim Acta* 1978;84:373–97.
15. Crilly RG, Jones MM, Horsman A, Nordin BEC. Rise in plasma alkaline phosphatase at the menopause. *Clin Sci* 1980;58:341–2.
16. Hodkinson HM. Calcium, phosphate and the investigation of metabolic bone disease. In: Hodkinson HM, ed. *Clinical biochemistry of the elderly*. Edinburgh: Churchill Livingstone, 1984:139–52.
17. Hodkinson HM, Bryson E, Klenerman K, Clarke MB, Wootton R. Sex, sunlight, season, diet and the vitamin D status of elderly patients. *J Clin Exp Gerontol* 1979;1:13–22.
18. Munan L, Kelly A, Petitclerc C. Population serum urate levels and their correlates. The Sherbrooke regional study. *Am J Epidemiol* 1976;103:369–82.

DISCUSSION

Dr. Meredith: Are you aware of any longitudinal studies looking at the rather complicated endocrine changes after the menopause?

Dr. Hodkinson: There are several such studies going on but none has yet come up with any clear answers. Such studies are certainly needed. In particular, we need to come up with better predictors of postmenopausal osteoporosis.

Dr. Guesry: You have dealt with only half the population. What about men? Do you think there is any need to treat elderly men with growth hormone and testosterone, as has already been suggested, or do you think this is unnecessary?

Dr. Hodkinson: I suspect this is unnecessary, but it depends on what the aim is. If we are talking about bone disease, the problem of osteoporosis is predominantly a female one. On any kind of cost-benefit equation we shall not do well if we start treating men with testosterone to prevent osteoporosis. However, this is certainly not the case for hormonal treatment in women. Osteoporosis in older women is an immense problem. If we could only predict those who are destined to suffer most severely, the cost-benefit equation would be highly favorable.

Dr. Nestel: What is your bottom line advice on hormone replacement in postmenopausal women? When one reads about this subject it appears that, as well as getting relief from menopausal symptoms, women on estrogens have half the coronary thrombosis mortality of those not receiving estrogens, quite apart from the beneficial effects on osteoporosis.

Dr. Hodkinson: I don't think it is yet possible to give definitive advice. However, we have to decide why we are giving hormone replacement therapy (HRT). Treatment is often given for the rather nebulous entity that is considered to be the menopausal syndrome. However, many of the symptoms ascribed to this have been shown to be more common *before* the menopause—headaches, for example. If replacement therapy is given with a view to preventing bone disease or vascular disease, we are talking about long-term treatment and I believe this to be quite onerous for the women who receive it. There is also the financial aspect to consider, apart from any possible risk of long-term replacement therapy (although I believe these have been exaggerated). My view is that we can afford to be very positive about HRT but we need to be highly selective in applying it.

Dr. Nestel: What do you mean by selective?

Dr. Hodkinson: We need to be able to identify groups of people whose risk is greater than average.

Dr. Nestel: So for the possible prevention of coronary heart disease, you would select only those women who have other risk factors for the condition?

Dr. Hodkinson: Yes, broadly. But one is looking at the osteoporosis problem as well. You need to combine the two: if you have high risk of either bone disease or ischemic heart disease the benefits of treatment of both are going to be very much better.

Dr. Chandra: Since the workshop is on nutrition, I wonder if you can speculate on the role of nutritional factors in modulating the hormonal changes you have described. Referring back to Dr. Guesry's question about HRT in males, we know that nutritional factors modulate testosterone levels so if we accept that in the elderly the frequency of nutritional deficiencies increases, then this may in part explain the lower testosterone levels. Testosterone is a very sensitive index of zinc intake, so even if only 20% of the population has marginal zinc deficiency in this age group, this could account for some of the differences in hormone levels. Is there any information to suggest that decline in estrogen output might be related to diet and nutrition rather than to primary gonadal failure?

Dr. Hodkinson: Decline in estrogen is a biologically programmed event. I don't think we can implicate diet in this. I accept that there are nutrients that may have an effect on the production of individual steroid hormones, but we are not talking about one estrogen. There is a plethora of estrogens and to determine whether zinc deficiency affects estrogen production you would have to measure them all—a daunting task and unlikely to yield a clear result unless there is a major effect. However, I think there is little doubt that there are interactions between hormonal status and dietary factors. Osteoporosis and osteomalacia are relevant examples. I am sure there are interactions in both directions.

Dr. Ballard-Barbash: Our National Cancer Institute has unearthed a number of studies that have examined the effect of dietary factors on estrogen metabolism. It has been postulated that several of these, including fat, alcohol, and fiber, have effects on estrogens. Early findings have confirmed effects on estrogen metabolism in several instances.

Dr. Durnin: It has been reported that exercise affects endocrine function in elderly men. Do you have any information on this?

Dr. Meredith: This also occurs in young men. Lower testosterone levels regularly occur in runners, and this is true for older men as well.

Nutrition of the Elderly, edited by H. Munro, and
G. Schlierf, Nestlé Nutrition Workshop Series, Vol. 29,
Nestec Ltd., Vevey/Raven Press, Ltd., New York © 1992.

Gastrointestinal Function in the Elderly

Barbara A. Bowman, *Irwin H. Rosenberg, and
†Mary Ann Johnson

*Department of Nutrition and Dietetics, Georgia State University, Atlanta, Georgia
30303, USA; *USDA Human Nutrition Research Center on Aging, Tufts University,
Boston, Massachusetts 02111, USA; †Department of Foods and Nutrition, University
of Georgia, Athens, Georgia 30602, USA*

It is commonly believed that intestinal function declines significantly with increasing age. Elderly people express gastrointestinal complaints more frequently than younger people and some disorders (e.g., diverticulosis, ischemic bowel disease) occur primarily in the elderly. In addition, most elderly people take medications, and many of these agents have significant effects on gastrointestinal function as well as on food intake.

Data collected during the first phase of the Georgia Centenarian Study illustrate the prevalence of gastrointestinal complaints with increasing age and their potential significance for nutritional status (Table 1) (1).

This chapter summarizes recent human studies of aging and the digestive system, emphasizing physiologic alterations associated with "normal" aging, particularly those that might affect nutritional requirements. Several comprehensive reviews are available (2–5).

ORAL CAVITY

Sensory changes in taste and smell and their effects on appetite and food intake are discussed elsewhere (see Murphy). Although stimulated salivary flow rates were not affected by age in the Baltimore Longitudinal Study of Aging (6), some medications may alter salivary flow. Decreased saliva production could increase the risk of dental caries and erosion. Whereas loss of teeth is common in current elderly cohorts (Table 1), secular trends in oral health suggest that tooth loss may not be universal in future cohorts.

ESOPHAGUS

Some minor abnormalities of esophageal motility (so-called presbyesophagus) have been described in elderly subjects. In the absence of neurologic disease (stroke,

TABLE 1. *Preliminary data on nutritional risk measures from the first phase of the Georgia Centenarian Study*[a]

	Age (yrs)		
	60–69 (n = 46)	80–89 (n = 44)	100+ (n = 19)
	% answering "yes"		
Do you now have an illness or condition that interferes with your eating?	13	14	26
Do you now have an illness that has cut down on your appetite?	4	5	5
Do you have trouble biting or chewing any kind of food?	17	16	37
Are there any kinds of foods that you don't eat because they disagree with you?	48	48	5
Do you wear dentures?	39	70	95
Have you had any spells of pain or discomfort for 3 days or more in your abdomen in the past month?	4	9	5
Did you have any trouble swallowing at least 3 days in the last month?	2	2	5
Did you have any vomiting at least 3 days in the past month?	2	5	0
Do you have any troubles with your bowels that make you constipated or give you any diarrhea?	17	25	37
Have you gained or lost any weight in the last 30 days?	11	7	11
Have you ever had an operation on your abdomen?	30	52	42
Have you ever been told by a doctor that you were "anemic" (had iron-poor blood)?	24	18	21
Do you smoke cigarettes regularly now?	16	0	5
In the past month, have you taken any medicines prescribed by a doctor?	76	74	74
In the past month, have you taken any medicines that were not prescribed by a doctor?	22	36	47
Are you on any kind of a special diet?	9	16	16

[a] Survey instrument of Wolinsky FD, Prendergast JM, Miller DK, Coe RM, Chavez MN. Preliminary validation of a nutritional risk index. *Am J Prev Med* 1985; 1: 53–9.
Participants are cognitively intact and community dwelling. For methods, see ref. 1.

diabetes mellitus), however, their clinical significance is uncertain and normal esophageal function appears to be maintained until at least 80 years of age (2,3,5). The effect of aging on gastroesophageal reflux does deserve study.

STOMACH

The most prominent effect of aging on gastrointestinal function involves the stomach. The prevalence of gastric atrophy and atrophic gastritis increases significantly

TABLE 2. *Effects of hypochlorhydria on nutrient bioavailability*

Nutrient	Bioavailability	Mechanism(s)
Calcium	Decreased	Decreased solubility
Iron	Decreased	Decreased solubility
		Decreased absorption of non-heme iron
Folate	Decreased	Decreased absorption
	Increased	Increased bacterial synthesis
Vitamin B_6	Decreased	Decreased digestion
	Increased	Increased bacterial synthesis
Vitamin B_{12}	Decreased	Decreased digestion and absorption of protein-bound vitamin
		Increased bacterial uptake

with age. In a survey of free-living Bostonians, the prevalence of atrophic gastritis increased from 21% of those age 60 to 69 years, to 31% of 70- to 79-year-olds, and to 37% of those older than 80 years (7). The physiologic consequences include reduced gastric acid secretion (hypochlorhydria, achlorhydria), decreased intrinsic factor secretion, and increased risk of bacterial overgrowth of the small intestine (reviewed in ref. 8).

Hypochlorhydria has several potential effects on nutrient metabolism, including reduced solubility and bioavailability of dietary calcium and iron, and reduced bioavailability of folate, vitamin B_6, and vitamin B_{12}. Interestingly, studies by Russell and coworkers indicate that a compensatory mechanism, increased bacterial vitamin synthesis, and intraluminal release of folate (9) and vitamin B_6, may prevent deficiency of these vitamins (reviewed in ref. 8). These effects are summarized in Table 2.

Work from the Goteborg Longitudinal Study has shown convincingly that low serum vitamin B_{12} concentrations are not a normal concomitant of aging but rather a consequence of gastrointestinal disease, particularly gastric atrophy (10). Healthy elderly subjects with normal gastric function and elderly subjects with atrophic gastritis absorb crystalline vitamin B_{12} normally; however, absorption of protein-bound vitamin B_{12}, which is reduced in atrophic gastritis, is normalized with antibiotic therapy (11). Nevertheless, covert small bowel bacterial overgrowth may be an underlying cause of malnutrition in the elderly. Treatment of 16 elderly patients with bacterial overgrowth resulted in significant weight gain and improvement in anthropometric measurements (12).

MOTILITY

Data on gastric emptying rates of the elderly are conflicting. In one recent study, gastric emptying of a mixed solid–liquid meal was significantly prolonged in elderly subjects: $t_{1/2} = 136$ versus 81 min ($p < 0.001$); however, there was no difference in mouth-to-cecum or whole gut transit time (13). In another study, using a liquid meal, the half-times for gastric emptying and small and large intestinal transit were not significantly different for young and elderly subjects (14). However, gastric emptying in the early phase (first 5 min) was significantly more rapid in the elderly (14).

In hypochlorhydria, gastric emptying should, in principle, be increased. A study of interdigestive motor activity demonstrated abnormal motility in all elderly subjects examined, independent of hypochlorhydria (15). Additional research is needed to establish whether and how hypochlorhydria and bacterial overgrowth affect gastric emptying and intestinal motility. Most studies indicate that age *per se* does not increase mouth-to-cecum transit time (16).

PANCREAS AND LIVER

With aging, morphological changes have been documented in both pancreas and liver. However, the functional significance of such changes is uncertain. Although stimulated pancreatic secretion of bicarbonate, lipase, and amylase was significantly decreased (by 40%) in older versus younger adults (17), digestive function appears to be maintained on usual dietary intakes, probably because of the excess physiologic reserve capacity. Similarly, whereas variable effects on hepatic drug uptake, metabolism, and clearance have been attributed to aging, liver function tests remain in the normal range, although the lithogenicity of bile is increased (18).

SMALL INTESTINE

Given the significant age-related decreases in average cardiac output (about 30%) and splanchnic blood flow (about 50%) (19), decreased intestinal absorption of nutrients might be expected in the elderly. In fact, absorption of fat, protein, and carbohydrate appears to be essentially unaffected by age in healthy elderly subjects, although high fat, high protein, and high carbohydrate meals are often less well tolerated.

For example, daily fecal fat excretion on a 100-g fat diet averaged 2.8 g, 2.5 g, and 2.9 g in subjects age 19 to 44, 45 to 69, and 70 to 91 years, respectively (20). However, at higher intakes (115–120 g), fecal fat excretion was significantly increased in elderly but not younger Swedish subjects (21). Interestingly, Southgate and Durnin reported a small difference in the apparent digestibility of fat, 96.4% versus 94.7% for young versus elderly women, on a fat intake of 80 to 95 g/day (22).

Most earlier studies of carbohydrate absorption relied on urinary recovery of nonmetabolized sugars. When the results of such studies are adjusted for decreased renal function (creatinine clearance), there is little evidence of carbohydrate malabsorption (reviewed in ref. 5). However, meals high in complex carbohydrate (up to 200 g) do evoke significantly higher breath hydrogen excretion in elderly subjects (23).

Milk and dairy products are often avoided by elderly people, who may associate them with gastrointestinal symptoms. Jejunal lactase activity does decrease with age, in contrast to sucrase and maltase, for which activities remain fairly constant throughout the life span (24). However, in a double-blind study, lactose malabsorption was not a predictor of symptomatic lactose intolerance in healthy elderly subjects (25).

In contrast, calcium absorption and adaptation to low calcium diets are significantly decreased in the elderly (26–28). Potential physiologic mechanisms include decreased gastric acid secretion, decreased skin synthesis of previtamin D, decreased renal activation of 25-hydroxyvitamin D, and perhaps end-organ resistance to 1,25-dihydroxyvitamin D (reviewed in ref. 29). In a recent study, a meal high in dietary fiber reduced calcium absorption in both healthy elderly subjects and elderly subjects with atrophic gastritis (30).

For some of the remaining micronutrients, including iron (31) and copper (32), there is little evidence of malabsorption in healthy elderly people. However, zinc absorption was significantly reduced in healthy elderly men (33). As discussed by Heseker (elsewhere in this volume), although cross-sectional surveys often report low blood vitamin concentrations in the elderly, vitamin supplementation usually normalizes blood levels, suggesting that dietary intake, rather than intestinal absorption, is inadequate.

Because intestinal lipoproteins are cleared more slowly in the elderly, older subjects actually have higher postprandial vitamin A concentrations after a test dose than younger subjects (34). Because of their high vitamin A stores, elderly Americans may have a lower margin of safety for this vitamin (35).

LARGE INTESTINE

Alterations in gastrointestinal motility may lead to constipation or diarrhea; both disorders occur in the elderly. Although clinical and patient definitions of constipation are often significantly different, it is clear that the prevalence of constipation increases substantially after 65 years of age and contributes significantly to morbidity (36,37). Because chronic constipation can be extremely refractory to treatment and may have a significant impact on the individual's sense of well-being, it is important to prevent this disorder by maintaining mobility and adequate fluid and fiber intakes.

CONCLUSION

There are age-related alterations in gastrointestinal function but they are usually not pronounced. However, even subtle alterations might increase the vulnerability of the elderly to illness and malnutrition, as discussed by Berry (elsewhere in this volume). Use of multiple medications, so common in this age group, and the presence of chronic disease significantly increase the potential for adverse effects on gastrointestinal function.

Gastric atrophy may have a significant effect on nutritional requirements for calcium and vitamin B_{12}, but efficient digestion and absorption of macronutrients (fat, protein, and carbohydrate) and most micronutrients seem to be maintained in healthy elderly people. Normative data, particularly for motility and intestinal transit, need to be established better for this age group.

ACKNOWLEDGMENT

We appreciate the assistance of Stanley W. Verhoeven, Reference Librarian, William Russell Pullen Library, Georgia State University.

REFERENCES

1. Johnson MA, Brown MA, Poon LW, Martin P, Clayton GM. Nutritional patterns of centenarians. *Int J Aging Hum Dev* 1992;34:57–76.
2. Altman DF. Changes in gastrointestinal, pancreatic, biliary, and hepatic function with aging. *Gastroenterol Clin North Am* 1990;19:227–34.
3. Shamburek RD, Farrar JT. Disorders of the digestive system in the elderly. *N Engl J Med* 1990;322:438–43.
4. Nelson JB, Castell DO. Aging of the gastrointestinal system. In: Hazzard WR, Andres R, Bierman EL, Blass JP, eds. *Principles of geriatric medicine and gerontology.* 2nd ed. New York: McGraw-Hill, 1990:593–608.
5. Rosenberg IH, Russell RM, Bowman BB. Aging and the digestive system. In: Munro HN, Danford DE, eds. *Nutrition, aging, and the elderly.* New York: Plenum, 1989:43–60.
6. Baum BJ. Evaluation of stimulated parotid saliva flow rate in different age groups. *J Dent Res* 1981;60:1292–6.
7. Krasinski SD, Russell RM, Samloff IM. Fundic atrophic gastritis in an elderly population. *J Am Geriatr Soc* 1986;34:800–6.
8. Kassarjian Z, Russell RM. Hypochlorhydria: a factor in nutrition. *Annu Rev Nutr* 1989;9:271–85.
9. Russell RM, Krasinski SD, Samloff IM, Jacob RA, Hartz SC, Brovender SR. Folic acid malabsorption in atrophic gastritis. Possible compensation by bacterial folate synthesis. *Gastroenterology* 1986;91:1476–8.
10. Nilsson-Ehle H, Landahl S, Lindstedt G, et al. Low serum cobalamin levels in a population study of 70- and 75-year-old subjects. Gastrointestinal causes and hematological effects. *Dig Dis Sci* 1989;34:716–23.
11. Suter PM, Golner BB, Goldin BR, Morrow FD, Russell RM. Reversal of protein bound vitamin B_{12} malabsorption with antibiotics in atrophic gastritis. *Gastroenterology* 1991;101:1039–45.
12. Haboubi NY, Cowley PA, Lee GS. Small bowel bacterial overgrowth: a cause of malnutrition in the elderly? *Eur J Clin Nutr* 1988;42:999–1005.
13. Wegener M, Borsch G, Schaffstein J, Luth I, Rickels R, Ricken D. Effect of ageing on the gastrointestinal transit of a lactulose-supplemented mixed solid-liquid meal in humans. *Digestion* 1988;39:40–6.
14. Kupfer RM, Heppell M, Haggith JW, Bateman DN. Gastric emptying and small-bowel transit rate in the elderly. *J Am Geriatr Soc* 1985;33:340–3.
15. Bortolotti M, Frada G, Vezzadini P, Bonora G, Barbagallo-Sangiorgi G, Labo G. Influence of gastric acid secretion on interdigestive gastric motor activity and serum motilin in the elderly. *Digestion* 1987;38:226–33.
16. Piccione PR, Holt PR, Culpepper-Morgan JA, et al. Intestinal dysmotility syndromes in the elderly: measurement of orocecal transit time. *Am J Gastroenterol* 1990;85:161–4.
17. Vellas B, Balas D, Moreau J, Ribet A. Exocrine pancreatic secretion in the elderly. *Int J Pancreatol* 1988;6:497–502.
18. Popper H. Summary—hepatologic problems in aging. In: Bianchi L, Holt P, James OFW, Butler RN, eds. *Aging in liver and gastrointestinal tract.* London: MTP Press, 1987:383–8.
19. Richey D, Bender A. Pharmacokinetic consequences of aging. *Annu Rev Pharmacol Toxicol* 1977;17:49–65.
20. Arora S, Russell RM, Kassarjian Z, Krasinski S, Kaplan MM. Evaluation of absorptive and hepatobiliary function in the aging digestive tract (abstract). *J Am Coll Nutr* 1987;6:434.

21. Werner I, Hambreus L. The digestive capacity of elderly people. In: Carlson LA, ed. *Nutrition in old age.* Uppsala: Almqvist & Wiksell, 1972:55–60.
22. Southgate DAT, Durnin JVGA. Calorie conversion factors. An experimental reassessment of the factors used in the calculation of the energy value of human diets. *Br J Nutr* 1970;24:517–35.
23. Feibusch JM, Holt PR. Impaired absorptive capacity for carbohydrate in the aging human. *Dig Dis Sci* 1982;27:1095–100.
24. Welsh JD, Poley JR, Bhatia M, Stevenson DE. Intestinal disaccharidase activities in relation to age, race, and mucosal damage. *Gastroenterology* 1978;75:847–55.
25. Rorick MH, Scrimshaw NS. Comparative tolerance of elderly from differing backgrounds to lactose-containing and lactose-free dairy drinks: a double-blind study. *J Gerontol* 1979;34:191–6.
26. Gallagher JC, Riggs BL, Eisman J, Hamstra A, Arnaud SB, DeLuca HF. Intestinal calcium absorption and serum vitamin D metabolites in normal subjects and osteoporotic patients. *J Clin Invest* 1979;64:729–36.
27. Ireland P, Fordtran JS. Effect of dietary calcium and age on jejunal calcium absorption in humans studied by intestinal perfusion. *J Clin Invest* 1973;52:2672–81.
28. Bullamore JR, Gallagher JC, Wilkinson R, Nordin BEC, Marshall DH. Effect of age on calcium absorption. *Lancet* 1970;ii:535–7.
29. Arnaud CD, Sanchez SD. The role of calcium in osteoporosis. *Annu Rev Nutr* 1990;10:397–414.
30. Knox TA, Kassarjian Z, Dawson-Hughes B, *et al.* Calcium absorption in elderly subjects on high- and low-fiber diets: effect of gastric acidity. *Am J Clin Nutr* 1991;53:1480–6.
31. Marx JJM. Normal iron absorption and decreased red cell iron uptake in the aged. *Blood* 1979;53: 204–11.
32. Turnlund JR, Michel MC, Keyes WR, Schultz Y, Margen S. Copper absorption in elderly men determined by using stable ^{65}Cu. *Am J Clin Nutr* 1982;36:587–91.
33. Turnlund JR, Durkin N, Costa F, Margen S. Stable isotope studies of zinc absorption and retention in young and elderly men. *J Nutr* 1986;116:1239–47.
34. Krasinski SD, Cohn JS, Schaefer EJ, Russell RM. Postprandial plasma retinyl ester response is greater in older subjects compared with younger subjects. Evidence for delayed plasma clearance of intestinal lipoproteins. *J Clin Invest* 1990;85:883–92.
35. Krasinski SD, Russell RM, Otradovec CL, *et al.* Relationship of vitamin A and vitamin E intake to fasting plasma retinol, retinol-binding protein, retinyl esters, carotene, α-tocopherol, and cholesterol among elderly people and young adults: increased plasma retinyl esters among vitamin A-supplement users. *Am J Clin Nutr* 1989;49:112–20.
36. Johanson JF, Sonnenberg A, Koch TR. Clinical epidemiology of chronic constipation. *J Clin Gastroenterol* 1989;11:525–36.
37. Castle SC. Constipation: endemic in the elderly? Gerontopathophysiology, evaluation, and management. *Med Clin North Am* 1989;73:1497–50.

DISCUSSION

Dr. Guesry: You mentioned that wheat bran reduces calcium absorption. It also reduces zinc absorption and I believe that the effect is not primarily due to the fiber but to the phytic acid that is very often linked with fiber in bran.

Dr. Kritchevsky: I was going to make that point too. It should also be pointed out that a high-fiber diet is not a low-fiber diet with added fiber. It is a diet where you have the fiber you get in the grocery, not in the pharmacy. Most studies have shown that on high-fiber diets or with high-fiber foods you don't generally see major effects on nutrient absorption unless the fiber is being consumed in enormous amounts. Study groups in the United States and Canada have concluded that fiber recommendations should be made in terms of grams per 1000 kcal, otherwise elderly people or children, who anyway eat smaller quantities of food, may erroneously be given excessive amounts on the basis that high-fiber diets are good, so more is better.

Dr. Bowman: However, it is virtually impossible to meet the US dietary recommendations for fiber intake without the use of foods that have been supplemented with fiber such as wheat bran. I agree that it is important to see whether there are physiological effects of adding fiber; it is also important to know whether these have biological or nutritional significance.

Dr. Kritchevsky: I'm not 100% convinced that the amounts of fiber that have been suggested are based on more than just a guess of what may be right.

Dr. Edwardson: Are there any examples of nutrients that are better absorbed with advancing age?

Dr. Bowman: Most studies have shown that there is a plateau of absorptive capacity that is maintained into old age. The possible exception to this is calcium. However, there is some suggestion that changes in intestinal membrane composition and fluidity may increase the absorption of fat-soluble nutrients, particularly vitamin A, in old age.

Dr. Heseker: Lipoproteins are increased in the blood of elderly people. Since retinyl esters are transported in the lipoprotein fraction, any differences in apparent vitamin A absorption in the elderly may be due to this difference in blood lipids.

Dr. Bowman: Studies on triglyceride clearance using stable isotope-labeled triglycerides support what you say and indicate slower intestinal lipoprotein clearance in the elderly (1).

Dr. Vellas: When we talk about gastrointestinal function in the elderly we must differentiate between elderly people in good health and elderly people suffering from anorexia and undernutrition. There is much greater modification of gastrointestinal function in the latter.

Dr. Munro: Is there any evidence that the rate of movement of cells on the intestinal mucosa slows down with age?

Dr. Bowman: In experimental animals, decreased rates of cell migration from the crypt to the villus occur in some species but not in others. In humans I am not aware of any studies. There is a suggestion that the villi may be somewhat shorter in the elderly but I have not seen any data on kinetics of intestinal cell maturation or turnover in humans.

Dr. Heseker: What is the prevalence of malnutrition caused by malabsorption in the elderly?

Dr. Vellas: It seems that malabsorption is not usually the cause of malnutrition in the elderly. Maybe the decrease in intake is a cause of malabsorption, but the aging gut *per se* is not a cause of malabsorption and malnutrition in healthy old people. When an old person has a poor food intake, then one of the consequences of the reduced intake is a decrease in gut function and possibly malabsorption. When we studied the physiological function of the gut in elderly people after starvation we found many alterations. Maybe this is the reason for the poor response to tube feeding that is usually found in old people.

REFERENCES

1. Krasinski SD, Cohn JS, Schaefer EJ, Russell RM. Postprandial plasma retinyl ester response is greater in older subjects compared with younger subjects. Evidence for delayed plasma clearance of intestinal lipoproteins. *J Clin Invest* 1990;85(3):883–92.

Nutrition of the Elderly, edited by H. Munro, and
G. Schlierf, Nestlé Nutrition Workshop Series, Vol. 29,
Nestec Ltd., Vevey/Raven Press, Ltd., New York © 1992.

Energy Metabolism in the Elderly

John V.G.A. Durnin

*Institute of Physiology, University of Glasgow, Glasgow G12 8QQ,
Scotland, United Kingdom*

In a discussion of energy metabolism in the elderly, we ought to try to be modestly precise about what exactly is meant by the "elderly." There is enough individual variation among a group of elderly people who are all of the same age to create difficult problems and if we lump together the whole age range from 65 years onward (as is frequently done in tables of energy and nutrient requirements), it is really impossible to be precise about anything. We should start therefore by subdividing our group of elderly people, and a minimum subdivision—and probably not an adequate one—is into two groups, one being the "young elderly," aged from 65 to 74 years, and the other the "older elderly," who are people 75 years or older. Almost certainly in a few years' time, when the number of really old people becomes considerably increased, we shall have to have a subdivision of the "older elderly" into people from 75 up to 84 years, and from 85 onward.

It may also be useful to have a categorization, independent of age, for elderly people who are free-living and those who live permanently in institutions (i.e., residential homes, long-stay hospital wards, or nursing homes for the elderly).

However, having made those suggestions, it will soon become apparent that the relative absence of definitive data makes it difficult to use any type of subdivision at all adequately.

FACTORS INFLUENCING ENERGY METABOLISM IN THE ELDERLY

There are several factors that might be anticipated to exert some influence on energy, but only some of them have any specific practical importance for the elderly. First, *energy expenditure* may be affected by (a) basal metabolic rate (BMR), (b) diet-induced thermogenesis (DIT) or the thermic effect of food (TEF), (c) physical activity, (d) mechanical efficiency of movement, (e) body weight and body composition, (f) body temperature, (g) sympathetic nervous system, and (h) muscle fiber type. Second, the *energy and nutrient intake* may be modified by (i) digestion and absorption, (ii) carbohydrate, fat, and protein metabolism, (iii) energy intake altered because of fiber intake, and (iv) low energy intake interfering with protein metabolism.

The physiological significance of these variables will be examined, not in absolute terms—such as whether DIT is important in influencing the level of energy expenditure—but in terms of whether the impact differs in old compared to young people.

With that premise, it is possible to speculate (with the aid of such experimental evidence as is available, together with some sensible physiological extrapolation) on the role of these various factors with regard to their influence on total daily energy expenditure. Since energy (and therefore food) intake is normally adjusted to equal, more or less, energy expenditure, energy expenditure is basically the most important factor affecting the nutrition of the elderly. Ways in which the eight variables listed above might modify energy expenditure in the elderly will now be evaluated. Poehlmann and Horton (1) have recently written a helpful review of some aspects of this topic.

Basal Metabolic Rate

The BMR represents the essential amount of energy required for the physiological functions of the body at complete rest (postabsorptive, thermally neutral, lying relaxed in bed, etc). All tables of BMR show a progressive reduction from birth up to old age, and this is sometimes given precise quantitative values, such as "a 23% fall during adulthood." Presumably this decrease reflects both a reduction in relative activity of many or most organs and tissues in the body together with an actual diminution in the mass of some of these organs and tissues. The skeleton and skeletal muscle are particularly obvious examples.

However, it is clear that much individual variability must occur in the reduction in BMR, and the data available, which consist almost entirely of cross-sectional studies, do not allow us to be at all exact if we are concerned with individuals or with special groups. It is probable that the reduction in BMR is more a reflection of changing body composition with age (e.g., more fat and less muscle) than in any real age-related alteration of metabolism. Elderly people, at least up to a moderately advanced age (70–75 years or so), who have avoided these changes in body composition may well show little decrease in BMR. This contention is supported by the data of Keys *et al.* (2), Tzankoff and Norris (3), and indeed by almost all of the classical data of Benedict *et al.* (4).

The result is that although recent data quoted in a report on energy and nutrient requirements in the United Kingdom (5), which included the scanty results collated by Schofield *et al.* (6) on the elderly, together with data on 101 men in Glasgow aged 60 to 70 years (Durnin and Choudhry, unpublished) and 170 elderly Italian men and 180 Italian women (Ferro-Luzzi, unpublished), demonstrate an overall reduction of between 10% and 20% between 30 years of age and 75 plus (Table 1), many individuals will not necessarily fit into this pattern.

TABLE 1. *Basal metabolic rate and age*

	Age (yrs)	Weight (kg)	BMR (kcal/d)
Men	30–60	74	1737
	60–74	74	1582
	75+	70	1405
			19% reduction
Women	30–60	64	1386
	60–74	64	1277
	75+	60	1212
			13% reduction

Body weights from ref. 17 and BMR calculated using formula in ref. 5.

Diet-induced Thermogenesis or Thermic Effect of Food

There is a certain amount of theoretical interest in discriminating between DIT and TEF, which is probably of minimal practical importance in man—certainly in the current context. They will be discussed here as if the terms were synonymous.

In certain situations, variations in DIT may have considerable long-term importance. For example, one factor conducive to the development of obesity might be a significantly low DIT, which usually amounts to about 10% of the energy available from the diet, and represents the energy involved in the processes of digestion, absorption, and metabolism. A low DIT means that proportionately less energy is dissipated in these processes and, over a lengthy period of perhaps many months or years, this small extra quantity might increase the likelihood of progressive fatness. However, the maximum difference from the average possible in a physiological state is likely to be no more than $\pm 2\%$ to 3% of total energy and is almost certainly of no significance for energy metabolism in the elderly.

Physical Activity

Physical activity is the variable likely to have most impact on differences in energy metabolism among elderly people. An excellent and extremely comprehensive review (quoting 1841 references!) of the varied aspects of physical activity in elderly people is contained in the book by Shephard (7).

Physical activity has many degrees of importance for the elderly. In simple nutritional terms, when physical activity increases, energy expenditure is also augmented and the energy required to replace that expenditure similarly becomes greater. Appetite will improve and the amount of food eaten is proportionately more. A secondary result of the increased intake of food is that there will also be a greater intake of nutrients—protein, minerals, and some vitamins. The activity itself results in improved muscle tone, more muscle and joint mobility, an extension of social contacts, and a general increase in the feeling of "well-being."

There is an obvious decrease in the overall level of physical activity with aging but it is a complex process, and the interindividual variability is enormous. There is a great deal of subjective and indirect information implying that, on average, there may be a significant reduction in activity from young adulthood onward. However, since the great majority of adults in the industrialized countries do not appear to be very active at any age (compare the average energy requirements of the population), this reduction may not be of a large degree. Despite the apparent widespread popularity of jogging, aerobics, and so forth, the jogging fraternity has a highly selected socioeconomic composition and there do not appear to be many socially or economically disadvantaged people who jog, nor a high proportion of elderly people. There is also, certainly in the United Kingdom and also in the United States, a definite ethnic bias.

Capacity for Exercise

There is a certain amount of physiological information on the diminution in the capacity for physical exercise that occurs with aging. The classical experiments of Dill (8) on his own ability to exercise throughout much of his adult life up to an age in the late 60s, and two Swedish studies (9,10), demonstrate clearly that there is a considerable fall in maximal exercise capacity, in cardiac output, in stroke volume, and in maximal heart rate with aging. Blood volume and total hemoglobin do not appear to change.

The importance of these reductions as far as energy expenditure is concerned is that the stress of physical exercise is often largely a function of its proportion of the maximal exercise capacity ($\dot{V}O_2$max). That is, if the $\dot{V}O_2$max is the equivalent of 15 kcal/min, then activity at a level of 7 kcal/min is quite tolerable. If the $\dot{V}O_2$max is 10 kcal/min, then an exercise at 7 kcal/min would be quite stressful. Therefore, elderly people with markedly reduced $\dot{V}O_2$max would be unlikely to undertake voluntarily any physical activity of more than rather light degree. However, improvement in the ability to exercise can certainly still be accomplished in the elderly. A monograph published by the WHO (11) gives illustrations of what can be accomplished by training: 10% to 15% increases in $\dot{V}O_2$max by men between 65 and 69 years, increases of 20% in vital capacity, improvements in lung diffusion, a lower systolic blood pressure, and greater strength. There may also be a considerable increase in the release of some of the adrenal and pituitary hormones.

Influence of Occupation

Occupation has an obvious relationship to physical activity, but is probably of little importance generally since most work situations in the industrialized countries do not require a level of physical activity that would be stressful to an average healthy elderly person. Therefore, the main influence of occupation might, paradoxically, be whether or not the degree of physical activity actually increased on retirement. Studies on this have been continuing in Nottingham, England, for some years (12,13) with no clear-cut conclusions. As one might expect, the variability is such that some men actually increased their activity levels after retirement, increased their muscle mass, and decreased their fatness, although the general picture was mostly in the opposite direction. Female factory workers almost universally became less active after retirement.

Influence of Degenerative Conditions

There is another feature of aging that may restrict physical activity, and that is the increased liability to suffer from one or more of the degenerative diseases of the circulatory and respiratory systems and particularly of the bones and joints. It might appear that many elderly people are not active because it is unpleasant, uncomfortable, or even painful for them to move around.

The proportion of elderly people who suffer from joint disabilities sufficient to incapacitate or inhibit movement is unknown and probably varies considerably for different countries, climates, occupations, and so forth. However, some informative data have been published in the United States (14) by the Department of Health, Education and Welfare. Table 2 shows the "normal" population, the remainder being "sufferers." However, it should be pointed out that never more than 1% of the group had a "severe" grade of the condition. The possibility arises, therefore, that degenerative arthritic changes may not be so important for most people in inhibiting physical activity.

The general conclusion may be that, whereas there is a negative relationship of aging to physical activity, up to 70 years or so the trend will often be rather gradual, and will be affected by the standard of health and by the amount of activity in the previous lifestyle.

TABLE 2. *Percentage of "normal" men and women related to those moderately disabled with arthritis of knees, hips, and sacroiliac joints*

Age (yrs)	Knees		Hips		Sacroiliac joints	
	M	F	M	F	M	F
35–44	98	98	100	—	99	—
55–64	92	89	97	96	96	99
65–74	86	75	94	96	98	98

TABLE 3. *Energy expenditure (kcal/min) of young and elderly men during standardized exercise*

Exercise	Elderly men	Young men
Arm ergometer 1	4.36	4.12
Arm ergometer 2	5.89	5.82
Treadmill 1	6.68	5.72
Treadmill 2	8.50	7.04

Mechanical Efficiency of Movement

The reduction in the efficiency of movement and in the control of balance that are part of the normal aging process have been described in several papers [summarized by Shephard (7)]. Our own study (15) gives a fairly typical set of results (Table 3).

We compared two groups, each of 12 men, one aged 20 to 30 years and the other 55 to 76 years. They were similar except for their age, all of them being unskilled laborers working in the construction industry. They performed two grades of standardized exercise involving arm work, and walked at two levels of standard exercise on the treadmill. The experiment was designed in the form of a Latin square to minimize the effects of fatigue and of other uncontrollable variables. There were no significant differences in either of the two arm exercises between the young and the elderly men, although the exercises involved moderate and moderately heavy exertion. In the walking exercises, the older men expended 17% more in the lighter exercise and 21% more at the heavier work load. The elderly men thus seemed to have similar degrees of mechanical efficiency to the younger men if the exercise did not involve much gross body movement, but the larger muscle groups and the control of balance required by walking resulted in a marked decrease in efficiency and an increased energy expenditure, presumably due to a general diminution of neuromuscular coordination.

Body Weight and Body Composition

Alterations in body mass with aging are not well documented. Most cross-sectional data show decreases in *height,* which may be as much as 5 to 7 cm for some groups between 30 and 70 years of age. This seems to vary considerably with socioeconomic group and with occupation—larger differences in height occur with aging in industrial communities compared to rural populations, whereas professional groups from the more privileged socioeconomic classes appear to show little change. Alterations in *weight* seem more complex and differ between sexes, so that men appear to have a slightly lower body weight at 65 to 70 years than at 40 years of age, whereas women frequently show an increase in body weight over this period. In general, in both the

United States (16) and in the United Kingdom (17), data show that weight increases with age and height decreases, with weight stabilizing around the age of about 70 years in men and then gradually decreasing due to the progressive loss of skeletal muscle and also, probably, fat. This is in general true for the average population of both men and women in each country.

Most of such data on body composition have been obtained from cross-sectional studies (18–21), although there is a small amount of good longitudinal information (22). Brozek (23) also described a redistribution of fat, there being proportionately less fat in the subcutaneous compared to the truncal sites in older people, which we have also documented (24).

The net result of a gradual increase of body weight up to a certain age in the elderly is that for any given amount and type of activity, *more* energy will be expended by the elderly compared to a younger group of adults.

Body Temperature

It is theoretically possible that energy metabolism might be influenced by a basic reduction in core temperature that might occur in advanced age due to a reduction in tissue metabolism, but this has not to our knowledge been documented.

Sympathetic Nervous System

The possibility that sympathetic nervous system activity increases with aging and may be influenced by diet and exercise has been well reviewed (1), but the evidence is inconclusive and difficult to analyze (for many reasons, including methodological problems). Its exact relationship to energy metabolism in the elderly is probably of limited practical importance in the current context.

Muscle Fiber Type

There seems to be a selective loss of type II fibers in the elderly muscle, which may therefore reduce the muscle glycogen stores and result in a diminished strength of contraction (25), although this may be more a reflection of lower levels of physical activity than a true aging phenomenon. However, despite this change toward failing function, muscle strength is still capable of improvement from an appropriate exercise program, even up to a very advanced age (26).

CONCLUSIONS REGARDING ENERGY EXPENDITURE

The conclusions that can be made about the overall effect of the various factors analyzed above on energy expenditure in the elderly are limited. First of all, for present purposes any important influence likely to be exerted by DIT, body temperature, sympathetic nervous system activity, and muscle fiber type can be largely eliminated. They are interesting to study but of little relevance here. *BMR* is possibly a major factor in reducing energy expenditure, especially over the age of 75 years. Alterations in *physical activity* may be of considerable importance and, in general, some reduction must almost certainly occur even before 70 years of age, although there will be large inter-individual variability and the state of health of the elderly person will obviously have much influence. *Body weight and body composition* are potentially able to affect energy expenditure, partly through changes in the fat-free mass but also because energy expenditure in any given activity is directly related to the cost of moving the body mass around. However, unless the alterations in body fatness (which is the variable that changes most) are fairly extreme, the final modification in energy expenditure may not be very marked.

The factor likely to have the major influence on average energy output will usually be physical activity, and therefore the way to prevent more than a minimal reduction with aging in total daily energy expenditure is to maintain an active lifestyle. Apart from the advantages of this for energy, there are the social, psychological, physiological and nutritional benefits to be obtained—greater physical mobility, increased social contacts, improved feelings of well-being, greater confidence, larger nutritional intake, increased bone density, and so forth.

MODIFICATIONS IN ENERGY METABOLISM RELATED TO INTAKE

Only brief mention will be made about topics under this general heading.

Digestion and Absorption of Nutrients

Another of the changes in function that is commonly believed to occur in the elderly, of some potential importance in nutrition, is relative malabsorption of foods. Good scientific evidence in favor of this is hard to come by. Southgate and Durnin (27) studied this as a by-product of assessing the energy values of protein, fat, and carbohydrate and measured, by chemical means and by bomb calorimetry, the total food eaten and the urine and feces excreted by groups of young and elderly men and women. The results showed no evidence of decreased efficiency of digestion and absorption with aging (Table 4).

Carbohydrate and Fat Metabolism

The proportions of carbohydrate and fat that supply the body with energy may have metabolic importance and could alter with aging, although no good evidence for this exists.

TABLE 4. *Percentage availability of "energy," protein, fat, and pentosan*[a]

Group	Energy	Protein	Fat	Pentosan
Young men	96.6	89.6	96.4	95.3
Elderly men	96.8	91.4	95.1	96.8
Young women	96.5	92.1	96.7	93.9
Elderly women	96.0	92.9	94.6	97.8

[a] From ref. 27.

Energy Intake Altered Because of Dietary Fiber

It is possible, but unlikely in the case of the elderly, that someone may have a large intake of fiber and a relatively small total intake of nutrients in the diet, with the result that the digestion and absorption of the nutrients are interfered with; this can sometimes be serious enough to result in malnutrition, with the availability of carbohydrate, fat, and protein in the food being reduced to the extent that the total net energy is inadequate.

Low Energy Intake Interfering with Protein Metabolism

The proportion of protein relative to the total energy in the diet may be within normal limits, but if the total diet is inadequate in supplying the energy requirements, the protein may be used as a source of energy and therefore be insufficient for the normal requirements of protein metabolism. Since this situation is potentially not uncommon in the case of elderly people—perhaps living alone, with a poor appetite, and little inclination to prepare adequate meals—minor degrees of protein malnutrition might be expected, especially in the older groups of the elderly. The relatively large studies in the United Kingdom (28) and the United States (29) that might have uncovered these cases if they existed did not appear to show much evidence of malnutrition, but distinguishing minor degrees of protein inadequacy is difficult. The condition may therefore be more common than is apparent.

ACTUAL ENERGY EXPENDITURES

Although there are published data showing that some elderly men have high levels of energy expenditure—more than 3000 kcal/d (30,31)—what is of more immediate concern is the proportion of elderly people whose energy expenditure is so low that the energy intake to supply that quantity will lead to insufficient intake of nutrients. Even in a younger group of the elderly, there must be some anxiety about the level of nutrient intake. For example, a recent study in the United Kingdom (32) found that the mean energy intake of men aged 50 to 64 years was almost exactly the same

TABLE 5. *Energy intake related to possible activity*

Energy intake of 60-yr-old woman = 1610 kcal/d
  Body weight = 66 kg
  ∴ BMR = 1290 kcal/d
DIT = 10% of intake = 160 kcal
  ∴ BMR + DIT = 1290 + 160
              = 1450 kcal
  ∴ Energy for all activity   = 1610 − 1450
                               = 160 kcal
  Housework (cooking, cleaning, etc.) costs approximately
  1 kcal/min above BMR
  2 h housework costs 120 kcal
  Remainder 160 − 120 = 40 kcal
Need to spend all remaining 22 h of day lying in bed.

DIT, diet-induced thermogenesis.

as that of men aged 25 to 34 years (2380 and 2440 kcal/day). The energy intakes of women of similar ages were also about the same (1610 and 1670 kcal/day). However, the actual level of intake of the women is surely a cause for some anxiety. An intake of 1600 kcal/day, when we allow for BMR and DIT, leaves such a small amount of energy for all the activities of the day that it implies an almost completely passive existence (Table 5).

Of even more concern is the proportion of these women who must be ingesting very low intakes of energy. If the mean energy intake is 1610 kcal/day, and the standard deviation is about 15%—a low-to-average percentage in these situations— about one-sixth of the whole population of women will have intakes between −1 and −2 SDs; that is, between about 1370 and 1130 kcal/day. These levels, if they represent the real situation, are surely indicative of a highly undesirable state.

It is clear that there is a considerable diversity of possible influences on energy metabolism in the elderly. This chapter has attempted to analyze their relative importance. We can do little to minimize the effects of some of these influences, but the one component capable of at least some modification in our daily life is physical activity. Its importance is surely great enough to warrant special consideration by all who are concerned with the present and future welfare of the elderly population.

REFERENCES

1. Poehlmann ET, Horton ES. Regulation of energy expenditure in aging humans. *Annu Rev Nutr* 1990;10:255–75.
2. Keys A, Taylor HL, Grande F. Basal metabolism and age of adult man. *Metabolism* 1973;22: 579–87.
3. Tzankoff SP, Norris AH. Longitudinal changes in basal metabolism in man. *J Appl Physiol* 1978; 45:536–9.
4. Benedict FG, Emmes LE, Roth P, Smith HM. The basal, gaseous metabolism of normal men and women. *J Biol Chem* 1914;18:139–55.
5. Department of Health. *Dietary reference values for food energy and nutrients for the United Kingdom.*

Report of the Panel on Dietary Reference Values of the Committee on Medical Aspects of Food Policy. London: HMSO, 1991.

6. Schofield WN, Schofoeld C, James WPT. Basal metabolic rate—review and prediction. *Hum Nutr Clin Nutr* 1985;39(Suppl):1–96.
7. Shephard RJ. *Physical activity and aging.* 2nd ed. London: Croom Helm, 1987.
8. Dill DB. The physiology of aging in man. The George Cyril Graves Lecture. Bloomington: Department of Anatomy and Physiology, 1961.
9. Åstrand PO. Physical performance as a function of age. *JAMA* 1968;205:729–33.
10. Saltin B, Grimby G. Physiological analysis of middle-aged and old former athletes: comparison with still active athletes of the same ages. *Circulation* 1968;38:1104–15.
11. Anderson KL, Masironi R, Rutenfranz J, Seliger V. *Habitual physical activity and health.* Copenhagen: WHO, 1978.
12. Patrick JM, Bassey EJ, Fentem PH. Changes in body fat and muscle in manual workers at and after retirement. *Eur J Appl Physiol* 1982;49:187–96.
13. Patrick JM, Bassey EJ, Irving JM, et al. Objective measurements of customary physical activity in elderly men and women before and after retirement. *Q J Exp Physiol* 1986;71:47–58.
14. Maurer K. Basic data on arthritis knee, hip, and sacro-iliac joints in adults ages 24–74 years. National Center for Health Statistics: Health and Nutrition Examination Survey. Washington, DC: US Government Printing Office, 1979.
15. Durnin JVGA, Mikulicic V. The influence of graded exercises on the oxygen consumption, pulmonary ventilation and heart rate of young and elderly men. *Q J Exp Physiol* 1956;41:442–52.
16. Abraham S, Johnson CL, Najjar MF. *Weight and height of adults 18–74 years of age.* National Center for Health Statistics: Health and Nutrition Examination Survey. Washington, DC: US Government Printing Office, 1979.
17. Rosenbaum S, Skinner RK, Knight IB, Garrow JS. A survey of heights and weights of adults in Great Britain. *Ann Hum Biol* 1985;12:115–27.
18. Noppa H, Andersson M, Bengtsson C, Bruce A, Isaksson B. Body composition in middle-aged women with special reference to the correlation between body fat mass and anthropometric data. *Am J Clin Nutr* 1979;32:1388–95.
19. Allen TH, Anderson EC, Langham WH. Total body potassium and gross composition in relation to age. *J Gerontol* 1960;15:348–57.
20. Forbes GB, Reina JC. Adult lean body mass declines with age: some longitudinal observations. *Metabolism* 1970;19:653–63.
21. Tzankoff SP, Norris AH. Effect of muscle mass decrease on age-related BMR changes. *J Appl Physiol* 1977;43:1001–6.
22. Robinson I, Dill DB, Tzankoff SP, et al. Longitudinal studies of aging in 37 men. *J Appl Physiol* 1975;38:263–67.
23. Brozek J. Changes of body composition in man during maturity and their nutritional implications. *Fed Proc* 1952;11:784–93.
24. Durnin JVGA, Womersley J. Body fat assessed from total body density and its estimation from skin fold thickness: measurements on 481 men and women aged from 16 to 72 years. *Br J Nutr* 1974;32:77–97.
25. Larsson L. Morphological and functional characteristics of the ageing skeletal muscle in man. A cross-sectional study. *Acta Physiol Scand Suppl* 1978;457:1–36.
26. Brown M, Rose SJ. The effects of aging and exercise on skeletal muscle—clinical considerations. *Topics Gerontol Rehabil* 1985;1:20–30.
27. Southgate DAT, Durnin JVGA. Caloric conversion factors. An experimental reassessment of the factors used in the calculation of the energy value of human diets. *Br J Nutr* 1970;24:517–35.
28. Department of Health and Social Security. Nutrition Survey of the Elderly. Report on Public Health and Medical Subjects, No 3. London: HMSO, 1972.
29. McGandy RB, Russell RM, Hartz SC, et al. Nutritional status survey of healthy noninstitutionalized elderly. *Nutr Res* 1986;6:785–98.
30. Durnin JVGA, Passmore R. *Energy, work and leisure.* London: Heinemann Educational Books, 1967.
31. Jerham VJ, Lavides BC, Durnin JVGA. A nutrition survey on crofters in North-West Scotland. *Nutrition* 1969;23:159–64.
32. Gregory J, Foster K, Tyler H, Wiseman M. *The dietary and nutritional survey of British adults.* London: HMSO, 1990.

DISCUSSION

Dr. Munro: If you were advising on recommended allowances for energy intakes at ages 65, 75, and 85 years, what would your figures be?

Dr. Durnin: A new UK report on energy and nutrient requirements has just been released (1). For the elderly we have suggested a blanket figure of 1.5 times the basal metabolic rate. This is equivalent to around 2000 kcal for men and 1800 to 1900 for women. Although this recommendation may in some instances be unrealistically high, we felt it better to overestimate the energy requirements of elderly people rather than to underestimate them.

Dr. Munro: In the abstract of a paper presented at the recent FASEB (Federation of American Societies for Experimental Biology) meeting in Atlanta (2), young adult men undertaking light activity had an average need of 3500 kcal per day based on double-labeled water. This is much higher that the predicted need of the young men (2900) given in the recent RDAs (3). What is your view, Dr. Durnin?

Dr. Durnin: There are two different methods involved in the double-labeled water technique for measuring total energy expenditure. One involves a relatively old-fashioned technique that has been used by geologists for years but produces accurate data. I am confident of the correctness of the results obtained using this technique. However, in recent years an automated mass spectrometry technique has been developed that in the hands of many people produces results that appear to be unreliable or systematically on the high side. These results seem just possible but are still much in excess of those that have been found in almost any other type of study. I have serious reservations in accepting that these results are valid.

Dr. Davies: We are used to thinking in terms of diminishing energy requirements with age and particularly with incapacity, but isn't it possible that energy expenditure may actually increase under these circumstances? I am thinking in particular of psychologically disturbed old people who are constantly on the move, and of incapacitated people struggling with crutches and frames.

Dr. Durnin: If you compare energy expended on a standard work load in people using these appliances, then it is higher than in people who are not disabled, but of course this does not mean that they are going to expend more energy overall because they will tend to limit their activities. Thus, I think it unlikely that there will be an increase in overall energy expenditure under these circumstances. I have no information on the psychologically disturbed but it is certainly possible that their energy expenditure is increased.

Dr. Ballard-Barbush: Are there any data on energy expenditure in Parkinson's disease?

Dr. Hodkinson: We have recently published work (4) showing that resting energy expenditure in Parkinson's disease in increased by about 25%.

Dr. Nestel: Is the reduction in resting metabolic rate with age largely accounted for by the reduction in fat-free mass or is it something more fundamental than this?

Dr. Durnin: There are few longitudinal studies. Brozek did one (5) where he followed men for about 30 years up to the age of 60 and found that he could explain the reduction in BMR almost entirely on the basis of changes in body composition, the more metabolically active tissues decreasing. On this basis there should be little change in BMR with advancing age if muscle bulk is retained by continued physical activity, and much of the loss of skeletal mass that occurs with aging could be prevented. However, there are only limited data on these points.

Dr. Berry: An increase in weight tends to occur after 60 to 65 years of age, at a time when there is a decrease in energy intake. Does this imply an even greater decrease in energy expenditure to account for the increase in weight, or is there a change in metabolic efficiency?

Dr. Durnin: The evidence that energy intake decreases much over this age range is rather slight. Most studies I am aware of that have compared 30-year-old and 60-year-old men have shown little change in overall intake, and sometimes a small increase with aging rather than a decrease. Thus, I don't think there is any need to invoke changes in metabolic efficiency. A difference in intake over expenditure of as little as 100 kcal per day over 10 to 20 years will lead to enormous differences in body mass.

Dr. Guesry: Is the 20% increase in energy expenditure during standard exercise tests in the elderly the result of obesity or is it due to muscular inefficiency or change in fiber type?

Dr. Durnin: We matched the groups for body mass so that their weights were the same. My explanation is that the difference is mostly due to reduced mechanical efficiency of movement, which is probably the result of reduced efficiency of balance, a common problem of aging. The small extra movements required to maintain balance probably account for the increased energy expenditure.

Dr. Merritt: Given the observation of a rather low total energy expenditure in the elderly, particularly in women, and a concomitant decrease in lean mass as a proportion of total body weight, what are the implications for dietary composition and nutrient density for the healthy elderly population?

Dr. Durnin: I find it difficult to accept the data related to energy intakes because these have generally been obtained under conditions that are quite at variance with normal lifestyles. I cannot believe that an intake of 1,600 kcal/day really represents the mean intake of a population of women aged between 50 and 65 years. I am not suggesting that the results are wrong, but I dispute that they represent the normal food intake over a long period of time. I prefer to work from the necessary energy expenditure and extrapolate upward to derive an adequate overall intake. If you take BMR plus the energy expended over the number of hours spent standing or sitting in the day, or walking around doing very little work, plus perhaps a small amount of moderate physical activity, you come up with a figure of about 1.4 times the BMR. Allowing 1.5 times the BMR in this group of women gives an overall intake of about 1,900 kcal per day, and this represents a very sedentary population. Thus, I should have thought that women aged about 65 to 70 years should aim at an intake of 1,900 to 2,000 kcal, and this would usually imply an adequate intake of all the different nutrients.

Dr. van Staveren: What practical advice can you give about the amount of exercise an elderly person should take? How do you derive the figure of 1.5 times the BMR?

Dr. Durnin: To get up to 1.5 times the BMR you need to have a minimum of about 2 hours walking moderately, not walking very slowly. This can be split up into different periods. Some people respond well to being told that they must walk for 2 hours every day. Others might respond better to general encouragement to be as active as possible.

REFERENCES

1. Dietary reference values for food energy and nutrients for the United Kingdom. Report of the panel on dietary reference values. Committee on medical aspects of food policy. London: HMSO, 1991.
2. Roberts SB, Heyman ME, Evans WJ, Fuss P, Young VR. The dietary energy requirements of young adult men, determined using the doubly labeled water method. *Fed Proc* 1991;5:A1647.
3. Subcommittee on the Tenth Edition of the RDAs, Food and Nutrition Board, Commission on Life Sciences, National Research Council, eds. *Recommended dietary allowances*. 10th ed. Washington, DC: National Academy Press, 1989.
4. Levi S, Cox M, Lugon M, Hodkinson M, Tomkins A. Increased energy expenditure in Parkinson's disease. *Br Med J* 1990;301:1256–7.
5. Brozek J. Changes of body composition in man during maturity and their nutritional implications. *Fed Proc* 1952;11:784–93.

Nutrition of the Elderly, edited by H. Munro, and
G. Schlierf, Nestlé Nutrition Workshop Series, Vol. 29,
Nestec Ltd., Vevey/Raven Press, Ltd., New York © 1992.

Undernutrition in the Elderly: A Physiological or Pathological Process?

Elliot M. Berry

Department of Medicine, Hadassah University Hospital, Jerusalem, Israel

Many studies have shown that there is a progressive decline in both energy intake and energy expenditure with increasing age, with alterations in body composition such that the proportion of adipose tissue increases at the expense of the lean body mass. Nutritional recommendations for the elderly are based on the assumption that these changes are detrimental. Thus, the recommendations have been designed in general to reverse the changes and restore the body composition and nutritional requirements to that of the younger age groups.

Other considerations suggest that this is not necessarily correct. Following the concept of Cannon that there is inherent "wisdom" in the body's metabolism and the comment of Shock that "aging is not a disease," the changes found in the elderly may in fact reflect their different physiological status and be an *adaptive* response designed to promote longevity. The aim of this chapter is to suggest that the "undernutrition" of the elderly—far from being a pathological process—may rather be an attempt to slow the progress of various disease processes, in particular atherogenesis and tumorigenesis.

ENERGY BALANCE AND BODY WEIGHT IN THE ELDERLY

The physiological changes in energy metabolism with increasing age have been studied by a number of workers. After the age of 30 years, energy intake decreases by approximately 12 kcal/day/year, and the basal metabolic rate (BMR) by 5 kcal/day/year (1). Height decreases by approximately 1 mm/year, and since the lean body mass (LBM) decreases by about 2% to 3% per decade, the BMR/metabolic mass remains relatively stable. There is also a decline of about 15% in total body water, together with a redistribution of body fat toward the trunk. Average body weight may not change over the decades and in fact decreases by 10% between the ages of 70 and 80 years. Body weight is considered to be a regulated variable and in view of the decrease in energy intake, there must be a corresponding decrease in energy expenditure (metabolic rate and physical activity). However, it is not clear which

TABLE 1. *Changes due to aging: physiologic function at 70 years as a percentage of that at age 30*

Cardiovascular system		Renal function	60
Cardiac output	70	Nervous system	
Maximum heart rate	75	Conduction velocity	85
Respiratory system		Resting glucose uptake	100
Vital capacity	60	Taste and smell	10
Residual volume	130–150	Metabolism	
Maximum O_2 uptake	40	Fasting blood glucose	100
Musculoskeletal		Basal metabolic rate	85
Muscle mass	70		
Hand grip, flexibility	70		
Bone mineralization	70–80		

is the cause and which the effect. Is the reduced LBM or metabolically active tissue responsible for the reduction in activity of the elderly, or is the reduction in LBM an adaptation to reduced activity and both consequent on a decline in energy intake? In other words, is the decline in food intake or the decline in energy expenditure the initiating factor? Measurements of energy expenditure in the elderly are not well documented (2), but activity rhythms in healthy elderly people are often well preserved (3). The RDA 1989 do not assume that a decline in activity is either desirable or inevitable. Rather, physical training, including strength training, is effective in the elderly and may blunt many of the physiological declines associated with aging (4). At all events body metabolism appears to become more "efficient" with increasing age, which would lead if unchecked to an increase in body weight that does not normally occur. Table 1 summarizes the function of various systems of the body at the age of 70 years as a percentage of that at the age of 30. In general, in the absence of disease, physical function continues to be appropriate but reserve capacity, the ability to respond to stress, diminishes linearly with time.

The decrease in appetite and weight loss with advancing age has led to a study of the neurophysiology of feeding behavior and has given rise to the term "anorexia in the elderly" (5), although it has absolutely no pathopsychological relationship to the disorder of adolescent girls. Brain levels of neuropeptide Y and norepinephrine, both stimulators of feeding, are reduced in Alzheimer's disease. The causes of a reduced body weight in the elderly are multiple and are detailed in Table 2. Most are related to organic, socio-economic, or iatrogenic (drug) causes. A percentage, not as yet known, may also be related to the physiological changes in metabolism detailed above and may thus be regarded as a normal response. The situation concerning fluid intake in the elderly is different and it appears that elderly people experience less thirst in response to water deprivation and must therefore drink more frequently (6). If the major causes of mortality in Western developed countries are heart disease (41%), cancer (22%), and strokes (8%), the principal causes of morbidity due to aging in the elderly are immobility and decreased cognitive function. For example, hip fractures start to rise in frequency after the age of 40 years, increasing exponentially, doubling every 6 years. We know virtually nothing about the causes

TABLE 2. *Causes of a reduced body weight in the elderly*

Normal physiologic changes with aging	Nutritional deficiencies
Decreased metabolic rate	Zinc
Decreased taste and smell	Secondary to alcohol
Conditions interfering with food intake	Psychosocial
Immobility, CVA; akinesia, Parkinson's disease	Depression
Chewing problems, dentition	Dementia
Manual dexterity, rheumatoid arthritis	Isolation
Systemic diseases	Financial
Chronic pulmonary and cardiac disease	Miscellaneous
Gastrointestinal problems	Drugs
Abdominal angina	
Cancer	

and prevention of the senile dementias that afflict 20% of people over the age of 80 years (7). However, all these processes may be influenced by the nutritional status of the patient.

THE EFFECT OF ENERGY RESTRICTION ON ATHEROGENESIS

Atheromatous plaques are multifactorial in origin, and their formation depends on genetic, metabolic, and environmental variables. With increasing age serum cholesterol increases as a result of increased production and diminished fractional clearance of low density lipoprotein (LDL). A wealth of epidemiologic evidence shows that atheroma increases with obesity, hypertension, diabetes, and hypercholesterolemia and that these diseases are both interactive and additive. Weight reduction, especially if coupled with physical activity, which increases high density lipoprotein (HDL) (8), is a primary (but not very successful) treatment for all these risk factors responsible for myocardial infarction and cerebrovascular accidents. Higher cerebral function depends on a steady supply of nutrients and oxygen. Brain organization is plastic, such that gradual ischemia of most regions may be accommodated without loss of function; in other words, if the same blood vessel was occluded over a number of months, instead of instantaneously as in a stroke, there would not be many neurologic sequelae. The problem of senile dementia is one of promoting and maintaining cerebral blood flow. Such changes may contribute to pathology in Alzheimer's disease, although the primary process is not vascular.

THE EFFECT OF ENERGY RESTRICTION ON LONGEVITY AND TUMORIGENESIS

More than 50 years ago McCay first documented that energy restriction in rodents increased longevity. It was also shown that underfed animals were less susceptible to experimental tumors. The findings are robust but there appear to be strain

TABLE 3. *Effects of nutrition on the incidence of mammary carcinoma in rats[a]*

Item	Dietary regimen		
	High fat ad libitum	Low fat ad libitum	High fat restricted
Energy intake (kcal/day)	41	41	34
Fat (g/day)	2.7	0.6	2.2
Linoleic acid (g)	1.5	0.3	1.2
Body weight (g)	217	190	182
Body composition			
Body fat	24	16	25
% protein	20	23	20
Tumor incidence (%)	73	43	7

[a] Adapted from Pariza, ref. 13.

variations—rats are more susceptible than mice. The putative mechanisms concern a number of systems, including the pituitary–adrenal axis, decreased gonadotrophins and enzyme induction, slowing primary aging processes (9), and protecting cellular homeostasis (10). The effects on the immune system are thought to involve decreased cell turnover and increased natural killer cell (NK) activity. Good and Lorenz (11) have examined these phenomena in genetically short-lived mice and in models of autoimmune disease. They have pointed out that the energy restriction is effective only if micronutrients (minerals, especially zinc, and vitamins) are present in adequate amounts, and its effect is enhanced by physical exercise (12).

The nutritional factors involve interaction between energy intake, energy content, and the dose of the carcinogen used. Total energy intake appears to be more important than the source of energy (13). The nature of dietary fat has been a major point of interest, since polyunsaturated fats may promote carcinogenesis while at the same time decrease the risk of atheroma. Pariza and coworkers have attempted to dissect the various interactions in a rat model, as shown in Table 3. It appears that the incidence of tumors depended on the total energy intake, the efficiency of utilization, and the circadian rhythm. It did not depend on the energy source, the percent of fat in the diet, the amount of linoleic acid ingested, body weight, or even on the age of introduction of the energy restriction. There may be an effect on free radicals, inhibiting an age-related increase in membrane 22:5 fatty acids, and thus causing a reduction in the peroxidation of membrane lipids (14). Peroxidized LDL lipids are more atherogenic than the native lipoproteins. Another possible mechanism is through modulating gene expression of metabolic enzymes and oncogenes (15). In animals, a restriction of 15% to 20% in food intake is effective in prolonging longevity and promoting resistance to tumorigenesis.

These findings have been confirmed in animals but have not yet been systematically applied to human geriatrics or oncology. Epidemiologic evidence in man is, however, supportive of a relationship between energy metabolism and carcinogenesis (13). Human obesity correlates with the incidence of carcinoma of the breast and uterus in women and prostate and colon in men. Carcinoma of the colon is associated with reduced physical activity, whereas increased exercise during adolescence lowers the subsequent risk of developing breast and uterine cancer. These findings suggest that research in the field of diet–cancer should concentrate more on the effects of total energy intake than on those of single nutrients, for example, fats, where neither breast nor colon cancer appears to be related to the quality of dietary fat ingested (16,17). In light of this argument, the appearance of cachectin or tumor necrosis factor (TNF) may be seen as an adaptive response to the presence of the tumor (18). TNF is secreted by cells of the immune system; it is cytotoxic/static to tumor cells *in vitro,* induces interleukin-1, and suppresses the principal enzyme responsible for storage of adipose tissue triglyceride, lipoprotein lipase. The other name for TNF, cachectin, emphasizes the anorectic potency of the protein. Thus, TNF aids the immune response and decreases caloric intake, which may help in tumor suppression.

THE EFFECTS OF ZINC ON THE PHYSIOLOGY OF AGING, BRAIN DEVELOPMENT AND FUNCTION, AND ON THE IMMUNE SYSTEM

Although we have considered the effects of total nutrition on longevity and tumorigenesis, the micronutrient zinc has a peculiar role in linking the different aspects of the physiology of aging, immunocompetence, and brain function. Zinc deficiency may lead to anorexia and a decrease in taste (hypogeusia). In the immune system there is decreased wound healing and T-cell dysfunction. Zinc supplementation alleviates the immune deficiency associated with acrodermatitis enteropathica (11). Zinc may also be involved in cerebral function in animals (19) and in man (20). Volunteer subjects given large doses of histidine develop "zincuria," cerebellar dysfunction, mental changes, and alterations in taste and smell that were all reversed by zinc replacement. Zinc is a cofactor in enzymes involved with myelination and in the formation of catecholamine and glutamate neurotransmitters. Thus, adequate zinc supplementation is a simple, practical recommendation for the elderly.

CHANGES IN BRAIN STRUCTURE AND FUNCTION WITH AGING

The debate over whether there is loss of neurons associated with the aging process has been summarized by Coleman and Flood (21). There appears to be decreased density of large neurons in the cerebral cortex and a decrease in cortical volume. Computed tomography (CT) studies on 64 healthy men aged between 31 and 87 years suggested that several brain regions are selectively altered with age—there is symmetrical atrophy of the cingulate gyrus and sulcus, with asymmetrical widening of the central and postcentral sulcus on the left and the intraparietal sulcus on the right (22). The functional correlates of these changes are speculative, but could relate to decreased verbal fluency and auditory tasks as well as to an age-related decline in the left-hand performance relative to the right. Positron emission tomography (PET) studies have not revealed any absolute changes in glucose utilization (23), despite the presence of structural atrophic changes, as shown by hypofrontality and the strong relationship between age and ventricular size as measured by CT. If structure–function relationships in the brain are analogous to other organs, then continued mental activity should be encouraged to counter the effects of brain atrophy.

Another attempt to assess brain function with aging used power spectrum analysis of electroencephalogram (EEG) waveforms from different brain areas during the performance of various neuropsychological–cognitive tasks (24). These were then correlated with a number of biochemical indices of nutrition. The principal findings from this study on 28 healthy subjects over the age of 60 years was a decrement in alpha wave activity in subjects with low thiamine levels. There were no correlates with zinc, perhaps because none was malnourished, but of interest was the finding that the EEG frequency responses of older subjects with high iron stores were similar to those of younger subjects; however, these studies are difficult to interpret because of the lack of consistency in the correlations between plasma iron, transferrin, and ferritin. It should also be noted that neuropsychiatric disorders due to cobalamin deficiency may occur in the absence of anemia or macrocytosis (25). Other studies in normal subjects over the age of 60 years showed a correlation between cognitive function and levels of vitamin C, B_{12}, folate, and riboflavin (26). Undernutrition may also suppress age-related changes in dendritic spines (27). Necropsy studies of human brains have shown an age-related loss of dopamine uptake sites in the putamen (28), which may explain the increased sensitivity to drug-induced Parkinson's disease with advancing age.

The effects of nutrition on brain function have not been fully studied in the elderly. The topic that was first investigated by Wurtman and coworkers at the Massachusetts Institute of Technology relates to the nutritional precursors of neurotransmitter synthesis, and to the competition between amino acids to cross the blood–brain barrier. Tryptophan competes with the other large neutral amino acids (LNAA), the concentration of which is in turn affected by the balance between protein (raises) and carbohydrate (lowers) in the diet. Older patients (over 40 years) perform poorly after carbohydrate meals as compared to protein, with lapses in sustained attention (29). Together with the Wurtman team and John Growdon at the Massachusetts General Hospital, we have recently investigated the effects of different diets on the action of L-dopa (another amino acid) in patients with Parkinson's disease. By using a suitable ratio of carbohydrate to protein, we were able to abolish postprandial alterations in the levels of the LNAAs and thus provide more predictable dose-response effects (30). Such simple dietary manipulations may be applicable to other neurotransmitter precursors and await evaluation for a possible role in improving cerebral function in the elderly.

CONCLUSION

It follows from the above discussion that active thin people should live longer and be less susceptible to cancer than age-matched subjects with the opposite habitus and lifestyle, but this remains to be proven. If trials are performed on energy restriction in the elderly, then vitamins, minerals, and trace elements (with particular attention to calcium and zinc) must be included in adequate amounts.

REFERENCES

1. Munro HN. The challenges of research into nutrition and aging. In: Munro HN, Danford DE, eds. *Human nutrition, Vol 6, Nutrition, aging and the elderly.* New York: Plenum Press, 1989:1–21.
2. *Recommended dietary allowances,* 10th ed. Washington, DC: National Academy Press, 1989.
3. Lieberman HR, Wurtman JJ, Teicher MH. Circadian rhythms of activity in healthy young and elderly humans. *Neurobiol Aging* 1985;10:259–65.
4. Smicklas-Wright H. Aging. In: Brown ML, ed. *Present knowledge in nutrition.* 6th ed. Washington, DC: International Life Sciences Institute, Nutrition Foundation, 1990:333–40.
5. Silver AJ. Anorexia of aging. *Ann Intern Med* 1988;109:890–904.
6. Phillips PA, Rolls BJ, Ledingham JGG, et al. Reduced thirst after water deprivation in healthy elderly men. *N Engl J Med* 1984;311:753–9.
7. Brody JA. Prospects for an aging population. *Nature* 1985;315:463–6.
8. Kannel WB. Nutrition and the occurrence and prevention of cardiovascular disease in the elderly. *Nutr Rev* 1988;46:68–78.
9. Masoro EJ. Food restriction in rodents: an evaluation of its role in the study of aging. *J Gerontol* 1988;43:B59–64.
10. Yu BP, Lee DW, Marler CG, Choi JH. Mechanism of food restriction: protection of cellular homeostasis. *Proc Soc Exp Biol Med* 1990;193:13–15.
11. Good RA, Lorenz E. Nutrition, immunity & cancer. *Nutr Rev* 1988;46:62–7.
12. Kritchevsky D. Influence of caloric restriction and exercise on tumorigenesis in rats. *Proc Soc Exp Biol Med* 1990;193:35–8.
13. Pariza MW. Dietary fat, calorie restriction, ad libitum feeding and cancer risk. *Nutr Rev* 1987;45: 1–7.
14. Langaniere S, Yu BP. Anti-lipoperoxidation action of food restriction. *Biochem Biophys Res Commun* 1987;145:1185–91.
15. Fernandes G, Venkatraman J, Khare A, Horbach GJMY, Friedrichs W. Modulation of gene expression in autoimmune disease and aging by food restriction and dietary lipids. *Proc Soc Exp Biol Med* 1990;193:16–22.
16. Berry EM, Zimmerman J, Peser M, et al. Dietary fat, adipose tissue composition and the development of carcinoma of the colon. *J Natl Cancer Inst* 1986;77:93–7.
17. Eid A, Berry EM. The relationship between dietary fat, adipose tissue composition and neoplasms of the breast. *Nutr Cancer* 1988;11:173–7.
18. Theologides A. Anorexins, asthenins and cachectins in cancer. *Am J Med* 1986;81:696–8.
19. Sandstead HH. Zinc: essentiality for brain development and function. *Nutr Rev* 1985;43:129–37.
20. Burnet FM. A possible role of zinc in the pathology of dementia. *Lancet* 1981;i:186–8.
21. Coleman PD, Flood DG. Neuron numbers and dendritic extent in normal aging and Alzheimer's disease. *Neurobiol Aging* 1987;8:521–45.
22. Andor T, Albert M, Stafford J, Kemper T. Symmetrical and asymmetrical changes in brain tissue with age as measured on CT scans. *Neurobiol Aging* 1990;11:21–7.
23. De Leon M, George AE, Tomanelli J, et al. Positron emission tomography studies of normal aging. *Neurobiol Aging* 1987;8:319–23.
24. Tucker DM, Penland JG, Sandstead HH, et al. Nutrition status and brain function in aging. *Am J Clin Nutr* 1990;52:93–102.
25. Lindenbaum J, Healton EB, Savage DG, et al. Neuropsychiatric disorders caused by cobalamin deficiency in the absence of anemia or macrocytosis. *N Engl J Med* 1988;318:1720–8.
26. Goodwin JS, Goodwin JM, Garry PJ. Association between nutritional status and cognitive functioning in a healthy elderly population. *JAMA* 1983;249:2917–21.
27. Moroi-Fetters SE, Mervis RF, London ED, Ingram DK. Dietary restriction suppresses age-related changes in dendritic spines. *Neurobiol Aging* 1989;10:317–22.
28. Allard P, Marcusson JO. Age-correlated loss of dopamine uptake sites labeled with [^{3}H]GBR-12935 in human putamen. *Neurobiol Aging* 1989;10:661–4.

29. Spring B, Maller O, Wurtman J, *et al.* Effects of protein and carbohydrate meals on mood and performance: interactions with sex and age. *J Psychiatr Res* 1983;17:155–67.
30. Berry EM, Growdon JH, Wurtman JJ, *et al.* A balanced carbohydrate: protein diet in the management of Parkinson's disease. *Neurology* 1991;41(8):1295–7.

DISCUSSION

Dr. Kritchevsky: The Lipid Research Clinics data show that in men, but not in women, a cholesterol below 170 to 180 mg/dl increases the risk of colon cancer. This is an area that has been bothering people for a long time and views range from dismissing the finding on the grounds that the affected individuals probably had cancer on entry to the program to saying it simply proves you should not worry about your cholesterol level. I think both views are wrong. If you have a high cholesterol you should lower it, but in some cases a low cholesterol may put people at risk of other diseases. Data are now emerging on body type and previous diet that may be relevant to this argument.

Dr. Berry: I have looked at adipose tissue biopsies in patients routinely coming for colonoscopy and have found no difference in the polyunsaturated/saturated ratio between cancer cases and controls, so I have been unable to confirm any effect of quality of dietary fat on development of colon carcinoma.

Dr. Harris: I want to make a comment about low cholesterol as well. There are data that show that people who have had prolonged weight loss drop their serum cholesterols and seem to be at increased risk of poor outcome. The issue to be considered is how much do we know about these individuals before they entered the studies? In some of the data we have examined from the National Center for Health Statistics there seem to be two groups of individuals with low cholesterols. One group has a very low risk of poor outcomes such as heart disease; the other has low cholesterol associated with poor health, and this group is at high risk of poor outcome. We need to segregate these two populations and look at them longitudinally to be able to identify any health risks associated with low cholesterol *per se*.

Dr. Schlierf: You recommended a low salt intake. Could you define this more precisely? We have already learned that the aging kidney is not able to conserve sodium, so sodium excretion will continue even if sodium intake is low. Orthostatic hypotension is one of the most common identifiable causes of falls in elderly people and this may be related to depletion of circulating blood volume due to sodium depletion. In addition, elderly people are often given diuretics that will aggravate the situation even more.

Dr. Berry: Salt intake will depend on the ambient temperature. If there is sweating, salt should not be restricted. My feeling is that, in view of the risks of fluid overload, hypertension, and heart failure in the elderly, salt intake should be moderate—only enough to give a little taste to the food. In my view, the problem of orthostatic hypotension commonly stems from overtreatment of hypertension in the elderly.

Dr. Chen: What is the possible mechanism to explain the change in tumor incidence induced by physical exercise?

Dr. Berry: I would guess that this is related to blood flow or to sympathetic activity.

Dr. Glick: Perhaps it could work through its effect on reducing obesity?

Dr. Kritchevsky: Exercise affects insulinemia, and insulin is a tumor growth factor. If you induce mammary tumors in rats and then make them diabetic, the tumor growth rate decreases significantly (1).

Dr. Schiffman: I should like to comment on food intake in the elderly. We did a large study (2) in a retirement home in North Carolina where we measured every ounce of food consumed and also collected 24-h recall data. The actual intakes were between 250 and 300 kcal greater than the recalled intakes, so recall is clearly inaccurate. The question still remains to be resolved as to how much these elderly people are really eating. I believe it is more likely that the weight loss occurring in old age is the result of absorption problems rather than undereating.

Dr. Berry: There is not much evidence for malabsorption in the elderly. If negative energy balance occurs, then they are either doing more exercise or eating less.

Dr. Bowman: Underreporting is an increasingly recognized problem in the use of 24-h recall. However, it is probable that such underestimates of food intake span the age ranges, so that even though the absolute numbers may not be correct, there may still be a relative change in old age.

Dr. Meredith: If you look at energy intake required for constant body weight in a metabolic ward, which is a fairly good measure of energy needs in the short term, there does not seem to be much change with age. From age 50 years to 80 it remains around 30 kcal/kg per day, although we know that during this period there is a reduction in lean mass. It thus seems that energy needs per unit body weight do not change much, although clearly per unit of lean body mass they may actually be increasing.

Dr. Berry: I am suspicious of metabolic experiments of this type in a free-living population. They are often done over weekends and who knows what happens then?

Dr. Mertz: There are many trace elements that are important for immune function and general health. The danger of recommending supplements for fortification is that we create imbalances. I hope I have interpreted your recommendation correctly in assuming that the nutrients you emphasize—zinc, calcium, and so on—should come from a balanced diet, not necessarily from individual supplements.

Dr. Berry: That is correct. However, I don't think there is any harm in giving vitamin supplements to the elderly since in most cases the excess will be excreted. Zinc may be involved in cerebral function in a number of ways. It is an endogenous modulator of glutamate neurotransmission, it is a cofactor of enzymes forming myelin and catecholamines, and it is involved in DNA repair. It is also involved in T-cell function.

Dr. Schiffman: One difficulty experienced by elderly people taking zinc supplements is that it is excreted in the saliva and causes an unpleasant taste. This leads to anorexia and poor eating.

Dr. Mertz: That is correct. There are other disadvantages such as the well known antagonism between zinc and copper.

Dr. Chandra: I agree that we should be cautious of giving zinc in excess . In studies that we published 7 years ago (3), we showed that if zinc intake exceeded 150 mg per day, there was a definite deleterious effect on a variety of immunological functions including neutrophil function and T-cell function. This may in part be because of its effect on copper absorption, but we also showed that serum and cell-bound lipoproteins increased, particularly the low density lipoproteins that are immunosuppressive. I think that when we refer to supplements as opposed to foods that are rich in zinc we have to be careful about the amounts, so once again the key word is moderation.

REFERENCES

1. Cohen ND, Hilf R. Influence of insulin on growth and metabolism of 7,12-dimethylbenz(A)anthracene-induced mammary tumors. *Cancer Res* 1974;34:3245–52.
2. Schiffman SS. Food acceptability and nutritional status: considerations for the aging population in the 21st century. In: Horisberger M, James P, Leathwood P, eds. *For a better nutrition in the 21st century.* Nestlé Nutrition Workshop Series, vol 27. Vevey: Nestec/New York: Raven Press; 1992 (in press).
3. Chandra RK. Excessive intake of zinc impairs immune responses. *JAMA* 1981;252:1143–6.

Nutrition of the Elderly, edited by H. Munro, and
G. Schlierf, Nestlé Nutrition Workshop Series, Vol. 29,
Nestec Ltd., Vevey/Raven Press, Ltd., New York © 1992.

Effects of the Aging Process on the Nutritional Status of Elderly Persons

Bruno Vellas

*Département de Médecine Interne et Gérontologie Clinique,
CHU Purpan-Casselardit, 31300 Toulouse, France*

Epidemiologic studies commonly demonstrate nutritional deficiencies in elderly populations (1,2). Surveys of independent community-dwelling elderly persons show that the consumption of minerals and vitamins are below the recommended daily allowance (RDA) for up to 50% of subjects, and that blood levels are subnormal in 10% to 30% (1). In nursing homes, 30% to 50% of the residents are substandard in body weight, midarm muscle circumference, and serum albumin concentration, indicating widespread protein-energy undernutrition (2). Blood levels are frequently low for both water-soluble and fat-soluble vitamins (2).

It is a major challenge to differentiate the effects of normal aging from manifestations of treatable disease. Since humans possess considerable reserve capacity beyond that necessary for ordinary needs, it is unlikely that aging *per se* causes malnutrition in the absence of associated disease or stressful events. Although social and behavioral causes are probably important, alterations in digestive and metabolic functions might also have an adverse impact on the maintenance of nutrition in elderly patients. Normal senescence causes a reduction in some physiological gastrointestinal functions. Recent studies have shown alterations in pancreatic and intestinal functions (3,4). Most of these studies have been conducted using animal models. Moreover, these changes still leave the average older person with a significant reserve capacity. In this chapter we will focus on three topics:

1. Is malnutrition inevitable in the elderly?
2. What are the patterns of malnutrition in the elderly?
3. What are the capacities of the elderly to adapt to starvation and refeeding?

IS MALNUTRITION INEVITABLE IN THE ELDERLY?

The Aging Process Study (APS) of New Mexico (5) provides unique information regarding the consequences of the aging process on the nutritional status of healthy elderly persons living at home by obtaining in-depth information about dietary habits and nutritional markers. The APS is a longitudinal study of the nutritional status of 304 free-living elderly persons. The methodology of this study has been described in previous publications (1). Nutritional intake is assessed during a 3-day period using a detailed diet record and subsequent computer analysis (1). Garry and associates found no important modifications between 1980 and 1989 in the nutritional status of the subjects from the APS (5,6).

Anthropometric and biochemical markers, as well as dietary intakes, remained relatively constant over the 9-year period in this healthy elderly population (5,6). Changes in energy intake could be accounted for by a reduction in basal energy expenditure due to the decrease in lean body mass, possibly associated with reduced physical activity with aging. Neither anthropometric nor biochemical nutritional markers showed significant alteration with age. The aging process alone had no important consequences on the nutritional status of healthy elderly people and the apparent requirements in this healthy elderly population seem to be near the requirements for young adults, with few modifications (7).

WHAT ARE THE PATTERNS OF MALNUTRITION IN THE ELDERLY?

Although the average older person will have an important nutritional reserve capacity, there will be considerable variation about the mean in any elderly population. With aging an increasing proportion of persons at the lower end of the distribution will pass beyond a threshold, possibly after periods of stress, at which time the reserve capacity will be depleted and may no longer satisfy the needs of that individual.

Patterns of Malnutrition in Independent Elderly People

Most of the important changes in nutritional status seen in elderly persons are secondary to one or more of many extrinsic factors such as diseases, medication, trauma, and living situation (8). One typical characteristic of older persons is the inability to recover completely weight lost due to a stress such as surgery. Progressive undernutrition often occurs without being diagnosed. Physicians need to look systematically at the nutritional status of the elderly patient. Periodic assessment of weight must be done. Incapacity and disability often cause anorexia. Forty percent of all patients receiving parenteral nutrition and 50% of all patients receiving tube feeding are over 65 years of age (9).

Patterns of Malnutrition in Nursing Homes

Although the high prevalence of both protein-energy and micronutrient deficiencies among elderly nursing home residents is generally acknowledged, there is no consensus on the relative contributions of the many possible causes for these conditions. Inadequate nutrient content in the diet (e.g., vitamin B_6) may play a role (10). A more important factor is decreased total intake, which may relate more to the underlying disease diagnosis of the patient than to his age *per se* (8). Some nursing home patients cannot eat unless someone feeds them, and there are frequently not enough staff to perform this service. Moreover, the struggle of nursing home patients to maintain their dietary intake is compounded by the catabolic effect of repeated infections.

ADAPTATION OF THE ELDERLY TO UNDERNUTRITION AND REFEEDING

Alterations in the adaptative response of intestinal and pancreatic function to starvation and refeeding might have an adverse impact on nutritional maintenance in elderly patients. Holt found that the proximal intestine responds to starvation and refeeding by abrupt variations in the numbers of villus epithelial cells and in enzyme secretion (3). We recently studied the exocrine pancreatic function of 15 older people with poor nutritional status in a geriatric medical service. We found an important alteration of the pancrealauryl test (4,11). These results are similar to those in a population of adults with chronic pancreatitis tested in the same laboratory. Similarly, we measured the plasma cholecystokinin (CCK) release after a liquid meal in healthy adult subjects and in two groups of aged people, one composed of undernourished subjects and the other of healthy, well nourished elderly persons. In the young adults CCK rose from 1 pM $\pm$ 0.4 (SD) to 3.5 pM $\pm$ 0.8. In the two distinct groups of aged subjects, there was no significant difference in basal CCK levels. However, the maximum CCK value was higher in the elderly group with undernutrition than in the healthy elderly group and the young adult group. These results suggest that the postprandial maximum level of CCK is not increased with aging but with undernutrition. Such alterations might have an adverse impact on nutritional maintenance in the elderly (4). Ciocon *et al.* (12) recently published an 11-month prospective study of 70 tube-fed patients age 65 to 95 years. Weight gain occurred in no more than 6% of the patients at any time in the study period. Only 5.9% showed increased albumin levels at the end of the study.

Although normal senescence seems not to have important consequences on the nutritional status of healthy elderly persons, the adaptation of pancreatic and intestinal function to starvation and refeeding can be disturbed. Unfortunately, there are only limited data available that are related specifically to the use of nutritional support therapy for elderly patients. Further research dealing with the many complex issues of providing nutritional support to the elderly is clearly needed.

CONCLUSION

In conclusion, the aging process is not a cause of malnutrition in a healthy elderly population. Active elderly and young controls are nutritionally not very different.

In contrast, the acutely ill, chronically ill, and dependent elderly people are notably less well nourished than either of the former groups. The requirements are different for these populations. Hence, RDAs based on age alone may be misleading and of little use to individual persons. An alternative approach may be to derive formulas for individualizing the adult RDA for each nutrient by including coefficients for such factors as age, the presence of specific diseases, and laboratory test results (7,13,14).

REFERENCES

1. Garry PJ, Goodwin JS, Hunt WC, Gilbert BA. Nutritional status in a healthy population: dietary and supplemental intake. *Am J Clin Nutr* 1982;36:332–9.
2. Rudman D, Feller AG. Protein-calorie undernutrition in the nursing home. *J Am Geriatr Soc* 1989; 37:173–83.
3. Holt PR, Kitler DP. Adaptative changes of intestinal enzymes to nutritional intake in the aging rat. *Gastroenterology* 1987;93:295–300.
4. Balas D. *Aging gut. Facts and research in gerontology.* New York: Springer 1991; (in press).
5. Vellas BJ, Albarede JL, Garry PJ. Diseases and aging: patterns of morbidity with age; relationship between aging and age-associated diseases. *Am J Clin Nutr* 1991; (in press).
6. Garry PJ, Hunt WC, Koehler KM, Vanderjagt DJ, Vellas BJ. Longitudinal study of dietary intakes and plasma lipids in healthy elderly men and women. *Am J Clin Nutr* 1991; (in press).
7. Vellas B, Albarede JL. Nutrient requirements of the elderly. *L'Année Gérontologique* 1990;4: 101–15.
8. Goodwin JS. Social, psychological and physical factors affecting the nutritional status of elderly subjects: separating cause and effect. *Am J Clin Nutr* 1989;50:1201–9.
9. Maslow K. Total parenteral and tube feeding for elderly patients: funding of an OTA study. *JPEN* 1988;12:425–32.
10. Sempos CT, Johnson NE, Elmer PJ, Allington JK, Methews ME. A dietary survey of 14 Wisconsin nursing homes. *J Am Diet Assoc* 1982;81:35–40.
11. Vellas BJ, Balas D, Lafont C, Senegas-Balas F, Albarede JL, Ribet A. Adaptative response of pancreatic and intestinal function to nutritional intake in the aged. *J Am Geriatr Soc* 1990;38:254–8.
12. Ciocon JO, Silverstone FA, Graver M, Cornelius JF. Tube feeding in the elderly patients, indications, benefits and complications. *Arch Intern Med* 1988;148:429–33.
13. Schneider EL, Vining EM, Hadley EC, Farnham SA. Recommended dietary allowances and the health of the elderly. *N Engl J Med* 1986;314:157–60.
14. Vellas B, Balas D, Albarede JL. Non reversible malnutrition in elderly people? *Age Nutr* 1990;1:67.

Nutrition of the Elderly, edited by H. Munro, and
G. Schlierf, Nestlé Nutrition Workshop Series, Vol. 29,
Nestec Ltd., Vevey/Raven Press, Ltd., New York © 1992.

Age-Associated Changes in Taste and Odor Sensation, Perception, and Preference

Claire Murphy

*Department of Psychology, San Diego State University,
San Diego, California 92120, USA*

When an elderly person observes that food simply doesn't taste the way it used
to, he or she is referring to food flavor. The chemical senses (taste, smell, and trigeminal sensitivity) all contribute to the perception of food flavor. The sense of taste
provides the individual with information about sweet, sour, bitter, and salty stimuli.
The sense of smell is extremely important for the perception of food flavor, since
the olfactory system carries the information about the many volatile substances in
food that add the nuances that transform, for example, a bittersweet substance into
a truffle, and a sweet and sour substance into a tangerine. The trigeminal system
provides the sensations of warmth, coolness, and pungency important to the perception of, for example, food flavored with chili peppers or mint.

Thus, in considering the effects of aging on "taste" or, more correctly, flavor, it
is essential to consider the effects of aging on olfaction and the trigeminal sense,
both for their own effects on appetite and dietary selection and for their contribution
to the overall constellation of food flavor.

TASTE

Many studies have reported that threshold sensitivity to taste stimuli declines with
age (see refs. 1–3 for reviews). Still to be definitively settled are the magnitude and
rate of the decline, the degree to which various taste qualities are differentially affected by age, and the role of threshold sensitivity in perception of real-world stimuli.

Suprathreshold taste intensity perception also shows a decline in the elderly, although the picture is less clear-cut (see ref. 1 for a review). Several investigators
have examined the psychophysical function for taste, that is, the function that relates
psychological intensities to the physical concentrations of a series of taste stimuli.
Enns *et al.* (4) found no alteration in the slope of the psychophysical function for
taste, that is, intensity grew with increases in concentration at the same rate, from
young adulthood to old age, although slopes for adults were less steep than for
children. Bartoshuk *et al.* (5) reported general stability of slopes in the elderly, and

attributed flatter slopes at threshold to lack of dental hygiene. Several other studies have reported some flattening of the slopes with age, further suggesting a decline in the ability of the elderly to track increases in a stimulus concentration (see ref. 2 for review). Most recently, Murphy and Gilmore (6) reported quality-specific age-related losses at the suprathreshold level. In a magnitude matching paradigm where subjects rated taste intensity against an outside standard, we found bitter to be the taste quality most affected by age, and sweet the least.

Because assessing taste intensity above threshold can be problematic in elderly subjects, we studied discrimination of suprathreshold taste stimuli using the Weber Ratio technique (7) and found the same pattern: older people showed greater impairment in discriminating bitter than in discriminating sweet.

OLFACTION

As mentioned above, perception of food involves not only taste information (i.e., information about sweet, sour, bitter, and salty), but also olfactory and trigeminal information from the myriad volatile components of foods and beverages. Independent of changes in sweet, sour, bitter, and salty perception, age-related differences in the constellation of volatile accompaniments to a taste may influence its perception, particularly its pleasantness.

Threshold sensitivity clearly declines with age, both for stimuli that are largely olfactory, and for stimuli that are largely trigeminal (see refs. 1–3 for reviews). Of importance for those working with food delivery to the elderly, those older persons who have developed Alzheimer's disease show significantly greater impairment in olfaction than the normal elderly, and the degree of impairment, at least at threshold, is related to the degree of dementia exhibited by the Alzheimer's patient (8). That this is a neurologically based phenomenon and not due simply to increases in nasal disease in the Alzheimer's population is quite clear (9).

Several studies have reported that suprathreshold intensity perception of olfactory and trigeminal stimuli is also significantly reduced in old age (10–12). In most cases the intercept of the psychophysical function was affected, in others the slope of the function.

Identification of odors is severely affected by aging (13,14), suggesting alterations in the overall quality perception of an odor. Furthermore, recent work in our laboratory shows significant age-associated loss of odor memory ability that is related to the sensitivity to, the familiarity of, and the identifiability of the odors (15).

FLAVOR PREFERENCE

Changes in flavor preference would be suggested by the changes in smell and taste function in the elderly. Several studies have addressed this issue. Laird and Breen (16) reported increased preference for tartness over sweetness in older subjects. Although Desor *et al.* (17) reported that 9- to 15-year-olds preferred greater sweetness and saltiness than did adults; they found no differences among adults up to 64 years old. Lack of information about the numbers of subjects falling into different adult age groups makes this result difficult to interpret.

Enns *et al.* (4) reported that college students had higher sucrose preferences (in aqueous solution) than children or elderly subjects. Dye and Koziatek (18) found that in older (65–88 years) nondiabetic subjects aqueous sucrose solutions became increasingly pleasant as concentrations increased over the range of 0.125M to 1M. Younger nondiabetic subjects rated 0.25M as the most pleasant and decreased their pleasantness ratings with each subsequent concentration. In adding salt to taste to chicken broth, older (36- to 66-year-old) subjects have shown higher salt preferences than younger (17- to 32-year-old) subjects (19).

Moncrieff (20) reported age-related shifts in preference for some odors. Simply being exposed to an odor (21) or to olfactory-taste mixtures (22) presented orally can produce shifts in pleasantness. Murphy (22) also demonstrated effects of context on the pleasantness of chemosensory stimuli. Since over the course of life the elderly have had significantly greater exposure than young subjects to both individual tastes and odors and to food and beverage systems, one might expect altered food and odor preferences in the elderly simply on the basis of exposure.

In addition, age-related changes in chemosensory perception also have the potential to alter preferred concentrations and hedonic judgments, since intensity is a powerful predictor of hedonic tone (23). For example, since the bitter function flattens with age, a stimulus which is too bitter for a young person might be less bitter, and thus more or less pleasant, for an elderly person.

The distinction between preference and pleasantness is an important one. Two useful measures of hedonics are the peak preferred concentration (i.e., the one concentration in a series that is chosen as the most preferred) and the pleasantness judgment (i.e., a kind of magnitude estimate of the pleasantness or unpleasantness of a given stimulus). These two measures provide different types of information concerning the hedonic quality of a stimulus. The former identifies the most preferred stimulus concentration in a series and the latter provides information about the pleasantness of each stimulus in the series. Both measures are important in assessing changes with age in pleasantness of tastes, smells, and flavors. For example, in a series of four concentrations of salt in a sample of vegetable juice, both young and old might choose the third concentration as the most preferred. However, the elderly might rate the fourth and highest concentration as pleasant whereas the young subjects might rate the saltiest stimulus as unpleasant. For this reason we have employed both of these measures in our studies of chemosensory hedonics over the life span.

We investigated the existence of age-related changes in preference in a sample of 300 people: 100 young adults, 100 middle-aged adults, and 100 older adults (24). We considered (i) whether the concentration most preferred in a series differs over the life span for salt, sugar, or citric acid stimuli; (ii) whether there are age-associated changes in pleasantness judgments for various concentrations of salt, sugar, or citric acid; and (iii) whether the background in which a stimulus is presented significantly affects the pleasantness of that stimulus.

The stimuli were sucrose, citric acid, and NaCl, each presented in four concentrations in deionized water and the same four concentrations in appropriate beverage bases. Degree of pleasantness or unpleasantness was measured on a bipolar line scale (22).

Pleasantness depended on age, background (beverage base or water), stimulus type, and concentration. Pleasantness ratings were less negative for elderly participants than for either young or middle-aged participants. Stimuli were judged less pleasant overall in water than in a beverage base, and concentration significantly affected ratings. Young and middle-aged participants found salt less pleasant than did elderly subjects. Overall, pleasantness ratings for sugar were higher for older subjects than for middle-aged, but not young subjects. High concentrations of sugar were also rated as more pleasant by the elderly participants than by the younger participants. Citric acid was less pleasant than NaCl for elderly subjects, but the reverse was true for young and middle-aged subjects.

Pleasantness judgments of all three stimuli were significantly affected by the background base in which they were presented. Sucrose and NaCl were both rated more pleasant in the beverage base, but the background produced greater differences in the pleasantness of NaCl than in the pleasantness of sucrose. The elderly rated salt higher than other participants did, regardless of its background. For all age groups, salt in water grew increasingly unpleasant when presented in increasing concentrations in deionized water. However, when presented in vegetable juice, both middle-aged and elderly raters preferred midrange salt concentrations. Ratings for sucrose produced inverted U-shaped functions. The elderly found the two highest concentrations of sucrose significantly more pleasant than the younger subjects did.

When peak preferred concentration was considered, analysis of variance showed significant differences as a function of background and of stimulus. Higher concentrations were preferred in beverage base than in water, suggesting the importance of studying stimuli in food and beverage systems.

This study has implications for dietary intake in elderly people, particularly those who must restrict their intake of salt and sugar. As a group, the elderly have an increased incidence of hypertension and diabetes. The elderly have decreased energy requirements because of lower energy expenditure. As a result, reduced intake is necessary to maintain energy balance. For older people who must restrict intake of salt and sugar for medical reasons, taste preference for these stimuli can have health consequences.

High concentrations of sucrose and NaCl were rated as more pleasant by elderly than by younger participants. The most obvious possible explanation for this effect is sensory, although this study was not designed to address the etiology of preferences. Older people may, for example, rate higher concentrations of salt as more pleasant simply because these concentrations are less salty to them than to younger subjects, who generally rate very high concentrations of salt as unpleasant. This sensory hypothesis follows from studies demonstrating some loss of suprathreshold intensity with aging for some of the simple tastants (6) and for amino acids (3). The results of the present study suggest that an experiment designed to test directly the ability of intensity to predict chemosensory hedonics across the life span would be worthwhile.

As with any cross-sectional aging study, the question of cohort differences in the present study arises. Environmental influences may have interacted with sensory influences on perception of flavor. The significant age effects on pleasantness ratings in the present study suggest the importance of longitudinal investigation.

Differential pleasantness depending on the background in which stimuli are presented suggests the importance of chemosensory elements other than taste in determining pleasantness. Age-associated changes in smell may be partially responsible for the differences in pleasantness judgments made by the young, middle-aged, and elderly subjects in our experiments. Previous experiments considering the ability of elderly and young subjects to identify blended food, with and without the sense of smell, clearly demonstrated that smell was more affected by the aging process than taste. An older person might, for instance, rate a stronger concentration of sugar in the beverage base as more pleasant, not necessarily because he desired more sweetness *per se,* but because he desired an overall stronger flavor. He or she could compensate for reduced sensory input from volatile components by increasing sweetness.

High concentrations of salt and sugar are more pleasant for older people than for younger people. The reasons for this may be cultural, contextural, or sensory.

Significant nutritional deficits in samples of elderly people have been reported (25). Whether these nutritional deficiencies result from decreased nutrient intake, from lowered rates of absorption and utilization (26), or from a combination of factors, is yet to be determined. We do know that up to 41% of elderly participants show deficient levels of serum protein, and 20% show deficiency in serum albumin (26).

RELATION BETWEEN SENSORY PERCEPTION AND NUTRITIONAL STATUS

Many of the recent studies of the chemical senses in aged people have been conducted with the implicit or explicit assumption that age-associated changes in chemosensory perception are related to health and nutritional status in elderly persons. Evidence to back this assumption is lacking. We sought this evidence in a series of experiments (27) in which we operationally defined nutritional status as the biochemical indices of total protein, albumin, and blood urea nitrogen (BUN).

We first investigated the effects of aging and biochemical status on preference for casein hydrolysate. We hypothesized that (i) older participants would find high concentrations of the amino acid mixture more pleasant than young participants would, and that (ii) participants with poorer biochemical status would prefer higher concentrations of casein hydrolysate than would those with better biochemical status.

To address these hypotheses, we tested 10 young adult and 10 elderly persons with a series of concentrations of casein hydrolysate: 0, 1, 2, 3, 4, and 5% w/v in an amino-acid–deficient soup base. Participants rated pleasantness or unpleasant-ness of the stimuli on the bipolar line scale described above. Venipuncture was performed on each person for assays of protein, albumin, and BUN.

Elderly participants had lower protein and albumin, and higher BUN values than young adults. The majority of the elderly, but only one young subject had low serum protein levels (defined as less than 6.5 g/dl). Analysis of variance (ANOVA) on peak preferred concentration (i.e., the concentration of casein hydrolysate most preferred by each participant) showed that elderly subjects preferred significantly higher con-centrations of casein hydrolysate than did the young.

Similarly, ANOVAs examining the effects of the three blood measures (grouped above and below the median) on peak preferred concentration indicated that higher concentrations of casein hydrolysate were preferred by those with higher values of BUN and those with lower serum albumin.

Since these results suggested an influence of age and biochemical status on the perceived pleasantness of casein hydrolysate, a major experiment was designed to investigate these variables further, as well as to determine the effect of perceived intensity on preference for casein hydrolysate. We hypothesized that higher con-centrations of the amino acid mixture would be preferred by older participants and those of lower biochemical status, and that perceived intensity would be predictive of preference.

Twenty young adults and 20 elderly persons performed magnitude matching to rate the intensity of the same six chemosensory stimuli used in the first experiment as well as of six auditory stimuli, included for matching purposes. The 40 participants also rated pleasantness of both auditory and chemosensory stimuli using the bipolar line scale described above. Blood was drawn and assayed as in the first study.

All three biochemical measures showed significant age effects. Compared to the young, elderly participants showed lower levels of serum protein and albumin, and increased levels of BUN. None of the young participants had low or deficient levels of protein, whereas a full 20% of the elderly had low serum protein levels (below 6.5 g/dl).

Elderly participants rated the amino acids as tasting significantly less strong than did young participants. Age group differences in intensity were similar at all con-centrations of casein hydrolysate: there were no differences in slopes of the psy-chophysical functions. Biochemical status was not significantly related to perceived intensity.

Age and blood status (as measured by the biochemical index described above) were significantly related to peak preferred concentration, but perceived intensity was not. Elderly participants preferred higher concentrations of casein hydrolysate than did young participants. Across age, participants with lower composite bio-chemical indices also preferred higher concentrations of amino acids. Thus, both older participants and participants with poorer biochemical status preferred higher concentrations of the amino acid mixture.

CONCLUSION

Because there is evidence to show age-related increases in olfactory and taste thresholds, one could argue that older peoples' preferences for higher concentrations of amino acids reflect impaired sensitivity. The present study suggests that the elderly participants' higher preferred concentration of casein hydrolysate is not simply due to generally lower perceived intensity. However, at lower concentrations, the individual flavor components of casein hydrolysate may fall below a person's odor or taste threshold and thus also alter its pleasantness. The importance of considering the complex chemosensory mixture when studying the effects of aging on taste perception should be clear.

ACKNOWLEDGMENT

The author's research and the preparation of this chapter have been supported by NIH grant No AG04085 from the National Institute on Aging.

REFERENCES

1. Murphy C. Taste and smell in the elderly. In: Meiselman EL, Rivlin RS, eds. *Clinical measurement of taste and smell.* New York: Macmillan, 1986:343–71.
2. Murphy C. Aging and chemosensory perception of and preference for nutritionally significant stimuli. *Ann N Y Acad Sci* 1989;561:251–66.
3. Schiffman SS. Age-related changes in taste and smell and their possible causes. In: Meiselman HL, Rivlin RS, eds. *Clinical measurement of taste and smell.* New York: Macmillan, 1986:326–42.
4. Enns MP, Van Itallie TB, Grinker JA. Contributions of age, sex and degree of fatness on preferences and magnitude estimation for sucrose in humans. *Physiol Behav* 1979;22:999–1003.
5. Bartoshuk LM, Rifkin B, Marks LE, Bars P. Taste and aging. *J Gerontol* 1986;41:51–7.
6. Murphy C, Gilmore MM. Quality-specific effects of aging on the human taste system. *Percept Psychophysiol* 1989;45:121–8.
7. Gilmore MM, Murphy C. Aging is associated with increased Weber ratios for caffeine, but not for sucrose. *Percept Psychophysiol* 1989;46:555–9.
8. Murphy C, Gilmore MM, Seery CS, Salmon DP, Lasker BP. Olfactory thresholds are associated with degree of dementia in Alzheimer's disease. *Neurobiol Aging* 1990;11:465–9.
9. Feldman JL, Murphy C, Davidson TM, Jalowayski AA, Galindo de Jaime G. The rhinologic evaluation of Alzheimer's disease. *Laryngoscope J* 1991;101.
10. Murphy C. Age-related effects on the threshold, psychophysical function, and pleasantness of menthol. *J Gerontol* 1983;38:217–22.
11. Murphy C. Cognitive and chemosensory influences on age-related changes in the ability to identify blended foods. *J Gerontol* 1985;40:47–52.
12. Stevens JC, Bartoshuk LM, Cain WS. Chemical senses and aging: taste vs smell. *Chem Senses* 1984; 9:167–9.
13. Murphy C, Cain WS. Odor identification: the blind are better. *Physiol Behav* 1986;37:177–80.
14. Doty RL, Shaman P, Applebaum SL, Giberson R, Siksorski L, Rosenberg L. Smell identification ability: changes with age. *Science* 1984;226:1441–3.
15. Murphy C, Cain WS, Gilmore MM, Skinner RB. Sensory and semantic factors in recognition memory for odors and graphic stimuli: elderly vs young persons, *Am J Psychol* 1991;104:161–92.
16. Laird DA, Breen WJ. Sex and age alterations in taste preferences. *J Am Diet Assoc* 1939;15: 549–50.

17. Desor JA, Green LS, Maller O. Preferences for sweet and salty tastes in 9- to 15-year old and adult humans. *Science* 1975;190:686–7.
18. Dye CJ, Koziatek DA. Age and diabetes effects on threshold and hedonic perception of sucrose solutions. *J Gerontol* 1981;36:310–15.
19. Pangborn RM, Braddock KS, Stone IJ. Ad libitum mixing to preference for salts in broths and sucrose in lemonade, compared to hedonic scaling. Sarasota, FL: Association for Chemoreception Sciences Annual Meeting, 1983.
20. Moncrieff RW. *Odour preferences*. New York: John Wiley, 1966.
21. Cain WS, Johnson F. Lability of odor pleasantness: influence of mere exposure. *Perception* 1978; 1:459–65.
22. Murphy C. Effects of exposure and context on hedonics of olfactory-taste mixtures. In: Kuznicki JT, Rutkiewic AF, Johnson RA, eds. *Selected sensory methods: problems and approaches to measuring hedonics*. ASTM STP 773. Philadelphia, PA: American Society for Testing and Materials, 1982:60–70.
23. Moskowitz HR, Kumraiah V, Sharma KN, Jacobs HL, Sharma SD. Effects of hunger, satiety and glucose load upon taste intensity and taste hedonics. *Physiol Behav* 1976;16:471–5.
24. Murphy C, Withee J. Age-related differences in the pleasantness of chemosensory stimuli. *Psychol Aging* 1986;1:312–8.
25. Gary PJ, Rhyne RL, Halioua L, Nicholson C. Changes in dietary patterns over a 6-year period in an elderly population. *Ann NY Acad Sci* 1989;561:104–12.
26. Yearick ES, Wang ML, Pisias SJ. Nutritional status of the elderly: dietary and biochemical findings. *J Gerontol* 1980;35:663–71.
27. Murphy C, Withee J. Age and biochemical status predict preference for casein hydrolysate. *J Gerontol* 1987;42:73–7.

DISCUSSION

Dr. Chen: Could the effects you showed be related to zinc deficiency?

Dr. Murphy: It was reported in the early 1970s that patients with loss of taste sensation could be improved by treatment with zinc (1). However, this finding was not confirmed in a double-blind study (2). Nevertheless, the notion that taking zinc will improve your taste has persisted in popular culture. In our taste and smell clinic we see many patients who have taken zinc for this reason but of the maybe 400 patients whom I have seen in the past few years, only two or three have reported that they improved on zinc. Thus, I think the chances that we are seeing an effect of zinc deficiency are very small.

Dr. Mertz: The connection between trace elements and taste function was first discovered in patients who were under copper therapy. The very first attempts to correct disturbed taste and smell thresholds were not made with zinc but with copper, which is just as effective as zinc. This strongly suggests that if trace elements are indeed involved in taste and smell function, certainly more than one is involved.

Dr. Meredith: In premenopausal women olfaction changes according to the estrogen status within the cycle. What happens after the menopause?

Dr. Murphy: The studies showing an effect of estrogen on olfaction only found the effect for certain kinds of odors. The cyclical effect was only captured by very complicated statistical analysis and it is certainly not a very large one. So far as postmenopausal effects go, the only studies that have separated men and women have shown that women preserve their sense of smell better than men.

Dr. Hallfrisch: Were your subjects screened for cognitive impairment or for smoking?

Dr. Murphy: We tested for cognitive function and it was well above average in the group as a whole. No one had cognitive impairment. So far as smoking is concerned, it is worth sketching in some of the background here. There have been two studies on aging and smoking that have to do with perception of bitter taste with advancing age (3,4). These showed that bitterness perception is compromised in older men more than in women, and this appears to be related to the fact that men smoke more. If this is a causal relationship it seems to be a cumulative one because acute studies in young smokers and nonsmokers show no difference in taste sensation unless a cigarette was smoked within 1 h of the test. The problem of retrospective analysis of smoking in a study such as ours is that it is difficult to define the problem among elderly individuals, some of whom may have smoked for 40 years but stopped 20 years ago, whereas others are current smokers but have only smoked for 10 years. In Southern California, defining smokers for these various studies has proved to be very difficult.

Dr. Guesry: You told us that there was no change in the sweetness threshold with advancing age. I assume your test was done using sucrose. Do you find the same with artificial sweeteners?

Dr. Schiffman: There is a big difference between natural and artificial sweeteners. The perception of the latter is considerably impaired in the elderly.

Dr. Glick: Did you find a correlation between impaired sense of taste and nutritional status?

Dr. Murphy: The results have been inconclusive. No one was overtly malnourished in our study population and among hundreds of people whom I have tested I can only think of a couple who had lost weight as a result of the problem.

Dr. Edwardson: Is there any evidence that old people use more added flavorings than young people?

Dr. Murphy: Yes, there is. One study done in 1983 (5) showed that older people added more salt to chicken than younger people. I have done similar studies and can confirm this, at least with respect to salt.

Dr. Edwardson: There is also the alternative possibility that adaptations occur over time. If you stop putting sugar on your cereal, after a few months the thought of eating cereal with sugar becomes unpleasant. Presumably such adaptations can occur in old age as well.

REFERENCES

1. Henkin RI, Patten BM, Re PK, Bronzert DA. A syndrome of acute zinc loss. *Arch Neurol* 1975; 32:745–51.
2. Henkin RI, Schechter PJ, Friedewald WT, Demets DL, Raff M. A double blind study of the effects of zinc sulfate on taste and smell dysfunction. *Am J Med Sci* 1976;272:285–99.
3. Kaplan A, Glanville E, Fisher R. Cumulative effect of age and smoking on taste sensitivity in males and females. *J Gerontol* 1965;20:334–7.
4. Smith SE, Davies PD. Quinine taste thresholds: a family study and a twin study. *Ann Hum Genet* 1973;37:227–32.
5. Pangborn RM, Braddock KS, Stone LS. Ad libitum mixing to preference for salts in broths and sucrose in lemonade, compared to hedonic scaling. Sarasota, FL: Association for Chemoreception Sciences Annual Meeting, 1983.

Nutrition of the Elderly, edited by H. Munro, and
G. Schlierf, Nestlé Nutrition Workshop Series, Vol. 29,
Nestec Ltd., Vevey/Raven Press, Ltd., New York © 1992.

Immune Response and Aging: Constitutive and Environmental Aspects

Alain L. de Weck

Institute of Clinical Immunology, University of Bern, 3010 Bern, Switzerland

Advancing age is accompanied by a decline of most cell-mediated and humoral immune responses, although the changes are sometimes selective and may appear to represent modifications in immune regulation (1). From all compartments and cells involved in the immune response, the thymus and T-lymphocytes appear to be the most directly affected, whereas monocyte, stem cells, and B-lymphocytes are less involved. Among the various immune phenomena detectable *in vitro* or *in vivo*, lymphocyte proliferation to mitogens, lectins, and alloantigens, the generation of cytolytic effector cells, delayed-type hypersensitivity, and primary and secondary antibody responses appear to be particularly diminished in the aged.

These changes do have an impact on disease and may be responsible, at least in part, for the increasing susceptibility of elderly individuals to infectious diseases, in particular tuberculosis and apparently acquired immunodeficiency syndrome (AIDS), for a lesser resistance to tumors, for changes in the manifestations of allergic hypersensitivity, and for the development of autoimmune diseases. It cannot be within the scope of this chapter to review all manifestations in which advancing age and changes in the immune responses have been implicated. I shall focus rather on the major cellular and molecular aspects of immunological senescence and on the external factors, such as nutrition, that may influence them.

Theories of aging can be classified broadly into two types. One type of theory states that aging is an orderly genetically programmed event that is the consequence of differentiation during growth and maturation (2). According to this type of theory, immune response cells have a limited proliferative and reproductive capacity that is genetically determined. This is also consistent with the observation of polymorphic immune aging patterns, as observed in various mice strains kept in a similar environment (3).

The other type of theory attributes aging to a progressive accumulation of faulty molecules resulting in cell dysfunction and death. This may be a stochastic event resulting from random synthetic errors, or from progressive damage due to environmental influences. In this case, adverse and environmental factors such as nutritional deficiency could well contribute to the manifestations of immunological aging.

HEMATOPOIETIC STEM CELLS AND DIFFERENTIATION OF IMMUNE COMPETENT PRECURSORS

The maturation of functional T- and B-cells from hematopoietic precursors is a prerequisite for a functioning immune system. Accordingly, the quality and quantity of the stem cells present in the bone marrow and the effectiveness of the aged environment to support stem maturation and differentiation should be evaluated. The total numbers of bone marrow pluripotent stem cells, characterized by their ability to form colonies in the spleen when transferred to lethally irradiated recipients, is unaffected by aging in most strains of mice (1). However, the proliferative capacity of these stem cells may be reduced in the aged.

Aging appears to affect more severely the committed stem cells of the lymphoid compartment and the maturational microenvironment of the bone marrow and thymus. The ability of the aged bone marrow to reconstitute immune responsiveness in irradiated young hosts has been the most common technique used for studying bone marrow aging, but recently new *in vitro* techniques have also been used. Early experiments using bone marrow reconstitution of irradiated hosts have suggested that age does not affect the production of B-cells and B-cell precursors. More recent work *in vitro,* however, has led to the conclusion that the aged bone marrow is not as effective as the young bone marrow in supporting B-cell differentiation. Mature B-cells, on the other hand, do not appear to be affected by aging in a major functional way.

Some studies indicate that although the total number of colony-forming cells in the aged bone marrow is not markedly diminished, the number of bone marrow T-cells and their ability to repopulate the thymus in irradiated animals decrease with age (1). As discussed in more detail below, the T-cell compartment appears to be markedly more affected by the aging process than the B-lymphocyte compartment (4). The ability of the aged thymus to serve as a site of T-cell maturation is possibly an important factor and thymic involution has been suggested to be the primary cause of immunosenescence. Although thymic function greatly diminishes with age, the number of peripheral T-cells does not change proportionately. This is in contrast to the situation arising after adult thymectomy, in which animals undergo a gradual decline in the number of T-cells, suggesting thereby that the aged thymus must retain considerable capacity for supporting peripheral T-cells. In the mouse, the capacity of the thymus to support the complete spectrum of T-cell differentiation is lost shortly after birth. However, even in old age, the thymic reticulum is capable of supporting some degree of T-cell differentiation. The role of thymic hormones in maintaining or generating functional peripheral T-cells is still not fully understood. However, several studies have shown that peripheral T-cell functions can be improved in aged animals by *in vitro* or *in vivo* exposure to thymic hormones.

In conclusion, the differentiation toward mature lymphocytes is defective in the aged animal, due largely to deficiencies in the maturation environment, and in part to loss of pre–B- and pre–T-cells in the bone marrow. This may lead in the aged individual to an accumulation of larger numbers of immature cells and/or of memory cells (1).

B- AND T-LYMPHOCYTE ACTIVATION

The generation of an immune response, be it cellular or humoral, requires the activation of antigen responsive T- and B-lymphocytes, and their entry into the cell cycle with subsequent expression of differentiated functions. The entry and transit of the cell cycle in T-cells require delivery to the cell surface of several signals triggering the sequential expression of several new proteins, such as the receptors for interleukin-2 (IL-2) and transferrin (5). Interleukin-2 is synthesized and secreted by specific subpopulations of T-cells. Interactions between IL-2 and its high affinity receptor are necessary to drive T-cells from the G_{1b} into the S-phase. The rate of cell cycle traverse appears similar in aged and young populations, but in older individuals a lower number of aged lymphocytes enters the cell cycle and in particular fewer undergo repeat cycles after stimulation.

Both T- and B-lymphocytes use similar intracellular mechanisms for transducing a membrane event into intracellular activation. Perturbation of some membrane antigen receptors, such as membrane IgM for B-lymphocytes or T-cell receptors for T-lymphocytes, leads to rapid activation of phospholipase C, which initiates the hydrolysis of phosphatidyl inositol, 4-5-phosphate. The products of this reaction, diacyl glycerol and inositol triphosphate, in turn activate protein kinase C and trigger the release of intracellular stores of calcium. A second major signaling mechanism involves the cyclic nucleotides cyclic adenosine monophosphate (cAMP) and cyclic guanosine monophosphate (cGMP), a system that appears to be a down-regulator of the first mechanism. Mitogen activation of aged T-lymphocytes is defective already at the earliest steps and problems can be identified at the levels of calcium mobilization, phosphatidyl inositol phosphate hydrolysis, and protein kinase C activation. Alterations in membrane composition and changes in the viscosity of the plasma membrane may also impair cell activation.

At a later stage, namely during transitions of cells from G_{1a} to G_{1b}, which includes the synthesis of several activation proteins, various defects have been clearly shown (5). Alterations in the generation of the proto-oncogene c-*myc*, in the synthesis of IL-2, and in the expression of IL-2 receptors have been reported (1). The synthesis of IL-2, a necessary second signal for driving T-cell entry into DNA synthesis, is low in both aged humans and experimental animals (6). The most significant factor controlling the quantity of IL-2 produced by aged lymphocytes appears to be the number of precursors. Whereas the amount of IL-2 produced per precursor cell is the same whether derived from an aged or young animal, the number of IL-2–producing cells is greatly reduced in aged individuals. Expression of the IL-2 receptor, which is synthesized and expressed during the late G_{1a} to G_{1b} portion of the cell cycle, is also deficient in aged animals. A decrease in the number of activated receptors per cell and a decrease in the number of cells expressing the receptors may

TABLE 1. *Cell cycle events affected by the aging process*

Cell cycle stage	Event	Changes with age
Go	Membrane composition	Lipid changes affect viscosity
	Membrane potential, ion	Na,K-ATPase activity decreases
	Cytoskeleton	Action polymerization changes
Go-G1a	Phosphatidylinositol hydrolysis	Decrease
	Protein kinase C activation	No change
	cAMP/cGMP	Controversial
G1a-G1b	Expression of new proteins	Low mRNA for IL2, IL2 receptor, GM-CSF, IL1, IL6, IFN-γ
	Expression of activation antigens	Low RL388, transferrin receptor
G1b-S	Lymphokine signals	Low DNA synthesis initiated in IL2R+ cells
G2M-G1	Cycle reentry	Impaired, accumulated chromatin damage, low DNA repair

both be responsible for the decrease in functional proliferation manifested by T-lymphocytes in aging. In addition, there seem to be some other defects limiting aged cell responsiveness to IL-2 at some site distal to receptor expression.

As far as B-cell activation is concerned, following activation with antigens or anti-μ reagents interactions with lymphokines also appear to be required for cell cycle transit and further differentiation (1). At least five T-cell–derived lymphokines have been characterized that influence B-cell growth and differentiation, such as interferon-γ, IL-2, IL-4, IL-5, and IL-6. Up to now, the effect of age on the synthesis and activity of these lymphokines has not been much studied. However, it has recently been shown by our group that messenger RNA levels expressed for a variety of lymphokines such as IL-1, GM-CSF, IL-6, and interferon-γ are also decreased in the elderly (6).

Several studies have indicated that subsequent cell cycles may be more significantly impaired in aged cells than the initial cell cycle, possibly in relation to alteration in chromatin structure and DNA repair mechanisms (1).

In summary, aged lymphocytes display a number of defects that prevent normal cell cycle entry and transit (Table 1). The inability of aged T-cells to enter and progress throughout the cell cycle is not due to a single defect but to a number of deficiencies. In addition to revealing multiple sites at which aging affects the activation sequence, the data available also indicate that only a portion of the lymphoid population is affected. Aged lymphocyte populations are a mosaic of normal active cells and of those that are defective.

AGE-ASSOCIATED ALTERATIONS IN CELL SUBSET DISTRIBUTION

The total number of B- and T-lymphocytes appears to be unchanged by aging, but changes in subset distribution may occur. Several studies in mice and man looking at the absolute numbers and proportions of T-lymphocyte subsets in aged peripheral blood lymphocyte populations have yielded conflicting results (1). A majority of the reports record a decrease in the proportion of T-lymphocytes, with a decrease in both CD4 and CD8 cells. However, the magnitude of the differences between aged and young populations is less than 20%, which is much less than the degree of functional decline that accompanies aging. A reduced number of functional receptors may also contribute to the ineffective triggering of aged lymphocytes. It must also be kept in mind that changes in T-lymphocyte subset distribution may not be a biomarker of aging but rather a reflection of some underlying disease processes. Indeed, selection of aged blood donors for good health, according to the so-called SENIEUR Protocol (7), indicates that a sizable proportion of the immunological decline phenomena usually attributed to age may in fact be due to additional non-age factors, such as environment (possibly nutrition) and disease.

IMMUNOLOGICAL REGULATORY CHANGES OCCURRING AS A FUNCTION OF AGE

Anti-idiotypic antibody production increases with age and is apparently responsible for the reduction in the amount of high-affinity antibody and the decrease in the avidity profile of antibodies produced by the aged. Downregulation by anti-idiotypic antibody seems to become much more important with age. The idiotype repertoire also apparently changes with age and the serum from aged animals is more efficient in suppressing antibody responses. Isotypic regulation, such as IgE regulation, may also be, at least in part, due to auto–anti-isotypic antibodies. We have accordingly started to investigate whether an increase in auto–anti-IgE antibodies may be responsible for the decrease in IgE-mediated allergic manifestations observed in the majority of elderly allergic patients (8).

Regulatory mechanisms mediated by suppressor cells are certainly also present in young and aged individuals. However, controversy remains regarding the role of suppressor cells in the diminished immune responsiveness of the aged. In the aged, several suppressor cell systems may operate. Regulatory T-cells control auto–anti-idiotypic antibody production and directly downregulate some responses but non–T-suppressor cells have also been reported (1).

One of the most intriguing aspects of immune senescence is the emerging data that indicate that aging does not equally affect all tissues and immune organs. In man, most of the data available for study of the immune functions are drawn from peripheral blood lymphocytes. However, several recent studies suggest that mucosal immunity, in particular the response in the gut-associated lymphoid tissue, is not markedly affected by age.

AGE, IMMUNE FUNCTION, AND DISEASE

Changes in immune regulation are apparently responsible for the increase in autoimmune phenomena and auto-antibodies that may lead, albeit not obligatorily, to specific organ or tissue injuries. Such changes in regulation are probably also involved in the age-associated decrease in manifestations of atopic allergy.

The age-related decrease in stem cell kinetics, differentiation, and functions may be critical to an effective response to stress, such as infection. Elderly patients with sepsis often fail to mount leukocytosis and to express fever, which are the result of lymphokine production.

The functional attributes of thymus-derived T-cells include delayed hypersensitivity reactions, production of lymphokines, killing of tumor cells, lysis of virus-infected cells, and transplantation rejection. In individuals above the age of 65 years, delayed cutaneous hypersensitivity reactions to ubiquitous recall antigens are reduced (9). Lymphopenia and anergy appear to have important prognostic significance in old age.

Of particular interest and beyond the genetic determinism of immune senescence is the recently formulated hypothesis that nutrition is a critical determinant of immune competence and risk of illness in old age (9). The fact that malnutrition in infants and children is directly associated with immune deficiencies is well documented. The impact of nutritional deficiency on the immune response is also evident from the phenomenon of acute anergy in patients undergoing severe trauma or operative shock, since this state of anergy can largely be overcome and abnormal immune response restored by nutritional supplementation.

In the elderly, nutritional deficiency may be more selective; in most instances it is probably not sufficiently pronounced to affect the immune response markedly. Very few studies have attempted up to now to correlate immune senescence with the state of nutrition or have attempted correction of nutritional deficiencies and their effects on immune responses in the elderly (9). In a group of apparently healthy individuals, those with clinical hematological and biochemical evidence of nutritional deficiency showed significant reduction in delayed cutaneous hypersensitivity reactions, in the number of T-cells, and in the lymphocyte response to phytohemagglutinin. Nutritional supplementation during a period of 8 weeks resulted in improved skin test responses, an increase in T-lymphocyte numbers, including the CD4 subset, and better lymphocyte proliferative response to phytohemagglutinin (10). In another study, prealbumin levels have been reported to correlate with impaired immune responses (11). Furthermore, nutritional supplementation appeared in a recent study to improve natural killer cell activity and mitogen-induced lymphocyte stimulation responses, to enhance delayed cutaneous hypersensitivity, and to increase IL-2 production (9).

Among the various nutritional elements, zinc appears to be particularly important since, on the one hand, the immune deficiency associated with low zinc diet is well documented, whereas on the other hand moderate zinc supplementation appears to improve delayed cutaneous hypersensitivity. However, megadoses of zinc, as well as of some other elements such as selenium, vitamin A or vitamin E, may also have immunosuppressive effects (9). Appropriate nutritional support may improve the response to immunization in the elderly, for example with influenza virus vaccine. It may also prevent postoperative complications, which occur more frequently and are more severe in elderly subjects who are malnourished. However, many more studies are required in order to assess more precisely the potentialities of nutritional supplementation in the elderly for improvement of their immune response and prevention of disease associated with immune deficiencies or dysregulation.

CONCLUSION

The combined effects of immunization, improved sanitation, better housing, and good nutrition have resulted in a dramatic decrease in childhood mortality and increase in life span in most industrialized countries. It remains to be seen whether improvement of nutrition in old age, possibly associated with a concurrent and increased stability of the immune responses at or near their optimal level, could be achieved in the elderly by the two pillars of prevention: optimum dietary intake and regular physical exercise.

REFERENCES

1. Thomas ML, Weigle WO. The cellular and subcellular basis of immunosenescence. *Adv Immunol* 1989;46:221–61.
2. Laughrea M. On the error theories of aging. A review of the experimental data. *Exp Gerontol* 1982; 17:305–17.
3. Kubo M, Cinader B. Polymorphism of age-related changes in interleukin (IL) production: differential changes of T helper subpopulations, synthesizing IL2, IL3 and IL4. *Eur J Immunol* 1990;20: 1289–96.
4. Makinodan T, Kay MMB. Age influences on the immune system. *Adv Immunol* 1980;29:287–330.
5. de Weck AL, Kristensen F, Joncourt F, Bettens F, Walker C, Wang Y. Lymphocyte proliferation, lymphokine production and lymphocyte receptors in aging and in various clinical conditions. *Semin Immunopathol* 1984;7:273–89.
6. Gauchat JF, de Weck AL, Stadler BM. Decreased cytokine messenger RNA levels in the elderly. *Aging Immunol Infect Dis* 1988;1:191–204.
7. Lighthart CJ, Corberand JX, Fournier C, Galanaud P, Hijmans B, Kennes B, Müller-Hermelink HK, Steinmann CG. Admission criteria for immunogerontological studies in man: the SENIEUR protocol. *Mech Age Dev* 1984;20:252.
8. Stadler BM, Nakajima K, Yang X, de Weck AL. Potential role of anti-IgE antibodies in vivo. *Int Arch Allergy Appl Immunol* 1989;88:206–8.
9. Chandra RK. Nutritional regulation of immunity and risk of infection in old age. *Immunology* 1989; 67:141–7.
10. Chandra RK, Joshi P, Au B, Woodford G, Chandra S. Nutrition and immunocompetence of the elderly. Effect of short-term nutritional supplementation on cell-mediated immunity and lymphocyte subsets. *Nutr Res* 1982;2:223–32.
11. Moulias R, Devillechabrolle A, Congy F, Wang A, Marescot MR, Lesourd B. Low prealbumin. A correlate of immunodeficiency in elderly patients. In: Chandra RK, ed. *Nutrition, immunity and illness in the elderly*. New York: Pergamon, 1985:165.

DISCUSSION

Dr. Chandra: I should like to make a couple of points. The first is that changes in immune responsiveness with age are not inevitable. There are individuals of 80 or 90 years of age who retain vigorous immune responses, as vigorous as those seen in young people. The second point is that in those elderly people who have nutritional deficiencies, defined by reduced dietary intake or by estimation of blood nutritional indices or some functional index of nutritional status, an improvement in nutrition is generally accompanied by an improvement in the immune response. In the population we have studied 25% to 30% of individuals, although apparently healthy and without evidence of significant systemic disease, showed evidence of reduced intakes and blood levels of various nutrients, particularly zinc, iron, vitamin C and β-carotene (1). We then provided a small supplement of these micronutrients that could be given to all persons in the group without the need to identify those who showed individual deficiencies. This supplementation improved *in vitro* lymphocyte reactivity, natural killer cell activity, and was associated with a significant reduction in common respiratory illness.

Dr. de Weck: It is important to stress the heterogeneity of the aging population. Many things can influence immune function and in any population of aged individuals there will be a wide variety of possible reasons for impaired immune responsiveness. Thus, without very large numbers of subjects followed up longitudinally, it will always be difficult to ascribe this or that change to this or that factor.

I should like to ask Dr. Chandra whether his supplementation study resulted in the reversal of anergy in old people as well as in improvement of lymphocyte reactivity.

Dr. Chandra: An improvement in skin hypersensitivity response was present but not statistically significant. However, we published a study in 1982 (2) in which we showed that anergy was reversed by diet treatment involving macro- as well as micronutrients after a period of 12 weeks in 7 of 14 individuals who were anergic at the start of treatment.

Dr. de Weck: I think that the anergy effect, or some measurable *in vivo* effect, will in the future be more important to study than *in vitro* assays, especially in patients submitted to surgical shock. It has been shown recently that patients who do not respond to intradermal injections of particular lymphokines have a much worse prognosis than those who are anergic but still respond to these lymphokines.

Dr. Schiffman: In one of our studies we found that there was an improvement in immune status simply as a result of improved food flavor. There was no difference in the amount of food or nutrients consumed, but the addition of odors and flavors seemed to improve the immune status. Could you comment on factors other than nutrition that may improve immunity?

Dr. de Weck: I have no data of this kind from our own studies.

Dr. Chandra: Stress is a very important factor that can affect the immune response to a variety of biochemical and other mediators. Perhaps by adding these pleasant odors to the diet there was a change in the overall satisfaction these individuals derived from their food and the happier state of mind produced may have affected their immune responsiveness.

Dr. Schiffman: Although we applied a "life satisfaction" scale, I do not think it was sensitive enough to pick up any differences resulting from these effects on the diet.

Dr. Guesry: It seems that nutrition plays a critical role in immunological function and the importance of trace minerals has been stressed. I think protein and long-chain polyunsaturated fatty acids also play a role that may be of considerable importance. I should like to ask Dr. Chandra whether he investigated such factors in those of his patients who had an incomplete response to trace nutrients.

Dr. Chandra: We did not do this in our study, but there is a large body of evidence to show the important immunomodulatory effect of lipids. There appear to be two considerations. The first is the amount of fat and the second, the type of fat. If in an animal model you feed more than 16% of the dietary energy as fat, you start to see an immunosuppressive effect that is more marked with polyunsaturated fatty acids. If you feed more than 40% as fat, the effect is much more marked and the distinction between polyunsaturated and saturated fats disappears.

Dr. Steen: Longitudinal studies of normal aging seem to show that the aging process becomes much more pronounced after the age of 70 to 75 years. Is this reflected in deterioration in immune function as well?

Dr. de Weck: It may be, and some data suggest that after 80 years there may be a very pronounced decline in immune responsiveness. But much of the available data do not include many subjects over the age of 80 and we need more information in the age range of 80 to 100 years.

REFERENCES

1. Chandra RK. Nutritional regulation of immunity and risk of illness in old age. *Immunology* 1989; 67:141–7.
2. Chandra RK, Joshi P, Au B, Woodford G, Chandra S. Nutrition and immunocompetence of the elderly. *Nutr Res* 1982;2:223–32.

Nutrition of the Elderly, edited by H. Munro and
G. Schlierf, Nestlé Nutrition Workshop Series, Vol. 29,
Nestec Ltd., Vevey/Raven Press, Ltd., New York 1992.

Energy Balance in the Elderly

Zvi Glick

*Department of Veterans Affairs, Sepulveda Medical Center, GRECC (11E),
Sepulveda, California 91343, USA*

Although the cut-off point is not clearly defined, and has great interindividual variability, age-related changes in energy balance of adults appear to be divided into two distinct, non-symmetric phases: the first phase is typically associated with a positive energy balance and an increase in weight and adiposity (but with a decrease in muscle mass), with more than 20% of the US adult population being overweight (1,2). This phase usually occurs between 20 and 65 years of age. The second phase, usually beginning after the age of 65 to 70 years, is associated with a loss of weight, mostly accountable for by a loss of lean body mass (3) (Fig. 1), and with a high prevalence of malnutrition (4).

The metabolic origins of the age-dependent compositional changes have not been clearly identified. Activity of growth hormone and testosterone, which promote lean tissue growth, is reduced with aging (5); this may contribute to the shift in balance from lean to adipose tissue. Indeed, growth hormone therapy can in part correct age-associated compositional changes (6). A decreased trophic effect of the autonomic nervous system on muscle and a decreased capacity for muscle fiber regeneration have also been implicated (7). Interestingly, with advancing age above 60

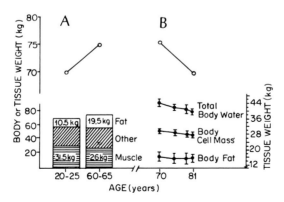

FIG. 1. Age-associated changes in weight and composition. **A:** Between 20 and 65 years. From Shepard JW (1). **B:** Between 70 and 81 years. From Steen B (3).

TABLE 1. *Age-related changes that may reduce energy intake and output*

Energy intake	Energy expenditure
Hypothalamic control	Basal metabolic rate ↓
Opioid feeding drive ↓	Protein turnover rate ↓
Senses	Protein turnover per kg lean body mass →
Sensory stimuli ↓	Na-K ATPase ?
Peripheral mechanism	Physical activity ↓
Insulinemia ↑	Thermic effect of meals ↓ ?
CCK ↑	Diet-induced thermogenesis ↓ ?

↓, decreased; ↑, increased; ?, unknown; →, unchanged.

years, mortality risk of being underweight becomes greater, whereas being mildly overweight is associated with the least mortality (8).

With aging a redistribution of body fat occurs, with gains in fat depots in the central and intraabdominal space, and away from peripheral subcutaneous fat. Such a redistribution is associated with increased risks of hypertension, diabetes, stroke, gallbladder disease, and coronary artery disease (9).

Understanding the age-related changes in energy balance requires a separate discussion of its two components: energy output and energy intake. Age-related changes that may reduce energy intake and output are listed in Table 1.

ENERGY OUTPUT: CONTROL AND AGE-RELATED CHANGES

Energy expenditure has been divided by nutritionists into the following components: (a) basal metabolic rate (BMR), (b) the thermic effect of meals (TEM), (c) physical activity, and (d) adaptive (diet-induced) thermogenesis (DIT).

Basal Metabolic Rate

BMR amounts to about 1400 to 1600 kcal per day, or 60% to 65% of total energy expenditure in a moderately active young adult (5). It originates primarily from, and therefore is highly correlated with, lean body mass. The metabolic origins of the BMR, especially the quantitative contribution of its individual components, are not clearly established. Protein turnover is thought to constitute about 15% to 25% of the BMR (10). The energy cost of the "sodium pump," needed to keep sodium extracellular and potassium intracellular against their concentration gradients, is estimated at 20% to 40% (11), and the cost of "futile" cycles in the metabolism of carbohydrate and fat are estimated at less than 5% (12). The energy costs of the other components of BMR—the maintenance of muscle tone and activity of involuntary muscles—have not been determined experimentally.

The BMR is governed by thyroid hormones that stimulate activity of the sodium pump (5), as well as protein turnover (5). In addition to its direct effect, T_3 can influence metabolic rate by enhancing sympathetic activity (13).

With advanced age there is a gradual 10% to 20% decline in BMR (14), which is typically accompanied by a reduced thyroid hormone activity (5) and a reduced responsiveness to norepinephrine (5). This decline also parallels the loss of muscle mass (Fig. 1). Of the known biochemical contributors to the BMR, only protein turnover is consistently reduced with aging (15), apparently reflecting the decline in lean body mass.

Thermic Effect of Meals

The TEM is the increment in energy expenditure that is observed upon meal taking and that lasts for several hours thereafter. The total energy of this thermic effect amounts to about 5% to 10% of intake. It has an "obligatory" component that reflects the metabolic cost of converting the ingested macronutrients into body protein, fat, and glycogen, and an adaptive component, which is stimulated by norepinephrine, and which apparently amounts to less than 30% of the total TEM (5).

The thermic responses to a glucose meal (16) and to a protein meal (17) are decreased with advancing age (but see ref. 18). One would not expect an effect of aging on the obligatory component of the TEM, but based on a reduced capacity for adaptive thermogenesis observed in old rodents (5), a reduced adaptive component of TEM in the elderly person is feasible.

Physical Activity

The amount of energy spent in physical activity varies greatly, with very highly active individuals expending more than 2000 kcal, and those moderately active expending 700 to 800 kcal, or about 30% of their total energy expenditure (5). Aging is usually associated with a significant decline in physical activity. In young subjects, as physical activity increases, there is a compensatory rise in spontaneous food intake, but data from animals suggest that older subjects do not adequately compensate intake for an increased expenditure, displaying a negative balance (5).

Aging is associated with a decline in physical working capacity ($\dot{V}O_2$max), amounting to about 5% to 10% per decade between the ages of 25 and 65 years (1,19). This decline is due to the smaller muscle mass, to changes in cardiac performance, decreased responsiveness to catecholamines, and other causes (19,20). A decline in physical working capacity means that a greater effort is necessary to carry out the same physical tasks. This will tend to cause a reduction in spontaneous physical activity, which will lead to a further decline in the capacity for work. Exacerbated by age-related diseases, such as cardiovascular disease, musculoskeletal disease, osteopenia, obesity, and others, a vicious cycle is created, which tends to limit physical activity and to reduce the physical working capacity. Physical training will correct age-related deterioration in physical working capacity by as much as 50% (21).

Physical training apparently potentiates the thermic effect of meals in both young and old individuals (18).

Diet-Induced Thermogenesis

Chronically overfed rats accrue only a fraction of the excess energy intake, while the rest is dissipated as heat. Clearly, a component of this heat originates from the additional metabolic costs incurred in depositing excess energy as fat (obligatory component), but in rodents, the major portion of DIT originates in the metabolically active brown adipose tissue (BAT) (22). Due to the small amount of BAT in man (5), the ability to dissipate of excess energy intake is apparently limited and difficult to demonstrate clearly (23). DIT in elderly persons has not been studied, but in rats the capacity for DIT (and for cold-induced thermogenesis) may decline with age to about 10% to 20% of the level found in younger animals (5). A decline in the capacity for DIT is compatible with lower tissue norepinephrine turnover (5) and a lower responsiveness to exogenous norepinephrine.

ENERGY INTAKE: CONTROL AND AGE-RELATED CHANGES

With age, there is a gradual decline in food intake that corresponds to the smaller energy expenditure. During the early decades of adult life, total energy balance is positive, whereas in the late years, especially among the institutionalized elderly (24), energy (and protein) deficiency becomes more common, as food intake often falls short of expenditure. However, whether a true "anorexia of aging" exists, independently of disease, medications, poverty, and psychosocial conditions that tend to suppress appetite, is not clear. Although as many as 30% and up to 60% or more of institutionalized elderly people display signs of energy deficiency, such signs were observed in only 3% of healthy free-living elderly persons (24). Moreover, no significant fat loss occurred in healthy elderly people between the ages of 70 and 81 years, only a small trend (3) (Fig. 1). I shall now present a brief overview of the control of feeding, highlighting age-associated changes that could influence feeding.

Central Control

The central control mechanism of feeding is a complex network of interconnected brain structures (5). The most studied anatomic sites are the ventromedial nucleus (VMH) and the paraventricular nucleus (PVN), the ablation of both of which leads to hyperphagia, and the lateral area (LH) of the hypothalamus, the ablation of which leads to aphagia. In addition to its proposed role as the center for the control of feeding, the hypothalamus is also a prime activator of the autonomic nervous system: the VMH activates the sympathetic branch and exerts an inhibitory effect on the parasympathetic branch of the autonomic nervous system (5) . Accordingly, VMH lesions stimulate vagal activity, hyperinsulinemia, and depletion of circulating substrates, leading to a state of overeating, whereas LH lesions stimulate sympathetic activity and substrate mobilization from fat and glycogen stores (autocannibalism) and induce satiety. The relative importance of a "feeding center" imbalance *versus* an "autonomic" imbalance in determining feeding behavior of hypothalamic lesioned animals has not been clearly defined.

Aging is associated with a significant decline in hypothalamic neurons in both the VMH and the LH regions (25). This could possibly influence the acuity of the sensations of hunger and satiety. Aging is also associated with a decline in activity of both the parasympathetic and the sympathetic branches of the autonomic nervous system (26), but their proportionate declines as pertaining to regulation of energy balance are not clear.

Neurochemical Mechanisms

The central control mechanism of feeding responds to cues from the periphery reflecting the nutritional state, as well as to sensual stimulation. Whatever effect a peripheral stimulus has on feeding, whether transmitted in the form of a metabolite, a hormone, or by a sensory input, is encoded into the brain neurotransmitter system to elicit a feeding response. These neurotransmitters include monoamines and neuropeptides.

Catecholamines

Direct injection of norepinephrine into the VMH or PVN will stimulate feeding, whereas its administration into the LH will inhibit feeding. This effect of norepinephrine is mediated through α-adrenergic receptors in the VMH and through β-receptors in the LH (5).

Aging is associated with a significant decline in catecholamine synthesis and activity in the hypothalamus, in both man and animals (25). In addition, brain tissue (studied in the cortex and cerebellum only) from aged rats has an impaired capacity for synthesis and regulation of α- and β-adrenergic receptors (27). A decline in catecholamine activity in the hypothalamus will also cause a suppressed release of hypothalamic gonadotropin-releasing hormone (GnRH), growth hormone–releasing hormone (GHRH), and thyroid-releasing hormone (TRH), leading respectively to impairments in reproductive functions, a decline in lean body mass, and a fall in BMR.

Neuropeptides

In the rat the administration into the hypothalamus of either opioid peptides or neuropeptide Y (28) will stimulate feeding, whereas the administration of corticotropin releasing factor (CRF) will suppress it.

It was reported that older rats respond less to opioid agonists or antagonists than younger rats (4), and that they have a lower concentration of opioid peptides in the hypothalamus (4). Aging may thus be associated with a decreased opiate-based feeding drive. CRF appears to play a role in the loss of appetite associated with depression (29), which is not an uncommon occurrence in the elderly. The orexigenic effect of neuropeptide Y is apparently not age-dependent (4).

Peripheral Control

Senses

Clearly, the extent of sensual pleasure that we derive from food influences food intake. With aging there is a decreased acuity of taste in association with a significant atrophy of the taste buds, and a reduction in the ability to detect odors and to identify the foods eaten (5).

Peptide Hormones

Peripheral injections of a variety of gastrointestinal hormones (and other peptides) into rats reduce food intake. These peptides include cholecystokinin (CCK), bombesin, gastrin-releasing peptide, glucagon, somatostatin, substance P, and neurotensin (28). However, the physiological significance of these hormones in producing normal satiety is not clear. A role for CCK in producing anorexia of aging was proposed recently on the basis that higher than normal serum levels of CCK were observed in elderly men, and that exogenous CCK-8 was more effective in decreasing feeding in older as compared to younger mice (4).

A continuous administration of insulin will suppress (unlike single injections that stimulate) feeding, perhaps by a direct effect in the brain (5). The importance of hyperinsulinemia in elderly feeding behavior is not known.

ANOREXIA OF AGING

Highlighted above are data on normal physiological changes in some aspects of the control mechanism of feeding that hold a potential for causing a downward trend in feeding during old age. However, the most common causes of anorexia found in elderly individuals (mostly institutionalized) are induced by disease states or they are psychosocial or poverty related (30,31). Common causes of anorexia in elderly people are given in Table 2.

Disease-Related Anorexia

Cancer: cachectin, interleukin, and prostaglandins produced in cancer patients are potent anorexic agents. Radiation therapy will impair feeding as well. *Chronic ob-*

TABLE 2. *Common causes for anorexia in the elderly*

Disease states associated with reduced food intake		Psychosocial causes
Cancer	Chronic constipation	Depression
Chronic obstructive pulmonary	Impaired mobility	Social isolation
disease	Dementia	Poverty
Swallowing difficulties	Depression	
Abdominal angina	Medications	

structive pulmonary disease: patients with chronic obstructive pulmonary disease may have difficulties in breathing and eating at the same time. *Swallowing problems:* elderly persons often develop swallowing difficulties related to cerebrovascular accidents, medications, and other disease states. *Abdominal angina:* stomach distension is accompanied by severe pain, leading to early termination of meals. *Chronic constipation:* leads to a sensation of fullness. *Medications:* digoxin and psychotropic and analgesic/anti-inflammatory drugs may cause anorexia in a large number of patients. *Dementia:* may produce an indifference to foods. *Depression:* will often produce anorexia, perhaps induced by an increased hypothalamic CRF. *Reduced mobility:* can result in an impaired capacity to obtain food and self-feed.

Socioeconomic Status

Social isolation and poverty will affect appetite and the ability to purchase desirable food.

CONCLUSION

Although there appear to be age-related changes in some components of the control mechanism of feeding, their significance for producing "anorexia of aging" remains to be determined.

REFERENCES

1. Shepard JW. Interrelationship of exercise and nutrition in the elderly. In: Armbrecht HJ, Prendergrast J, Coe R, eds. *Nutritional intervention in the aging process.* New York: Springer–Verlag, 1984: 315–31.
2. Van Italie TB. The problem of obesity. Health implications of overweight and obesity in the United States. *Ann Intern Med* 1985;103:983–8.
3. Steen B. Body composition and aging. *Nutr Rev* 1988;46:45–51.
4. Morley JE, Silver AJ. Anorexia in the elderly. *Neurobiol Aging* 1988;9:9–16.
5. Glick Z. Energy balance. In: Morley JE, Glick Z, Rubenstein LZ, eds. *Geriatric nutrition.* New York: Raven Press, 1990:27–40.
6. Rudman D, Feller AG, Nagraj HS, *et al.* Effect of human growth hormone in men over 60 years old. *N Engl J Med* 1990;323:1–6.

7. Evans WJ. Exercise and muscle metabolism in the elderly. In: Hutchinson ML, Munro HN, eds. *Nutrition and aging.* New York: Academic Press, 1986:179–91.
8. Andres R. Mortality and obesity: the rationale for age-specific height-weight tables. In: Andres R, Bierman EL, Hazzard WR, eds. *Principles of geriatric medicine.* New York: McGraw-Hill, 1985: 311–8.
9. Schwartz RS, Shuman WP, Bradbury VL, *et al.* Body fat distribution in healthy young and old men. *J Gerontol* 1990;45:M181–5.
10. Waterlow JC, Garlick PJ, Millward DJ. *Protein turnover in mammalian tissues and in the whole body.* New York: Elsevier, North Holland, 1978.
11. Milligan LP, McBride BW. Energy cost of ion pumping by animal tissues. *J Nutr* 1985;115:1374–82.
12. Himms-Hagen J. Cellular thermogenesis. *Annu Rev Physiol* 1976;38:315–51.
13. Rothwell NJ, Saville ME, Stock MJ. Sympathetic and thyroid influences on metabolic rate in fed, fasted, and refed rats. *Am J Physiol* 1982;243:R339–46.
14. Chernoff R, Lipschitz DA. Nutrition and aging. In: Shills M, Young V, eds. *Modern nutrition in health and disease.* 7th ed. Philadelphia: Lea and Febiger, 1988:982–1000.
15. Young VR. Impact of aging on protein metabolism. In: Ambrecht HJ, Prendergast JM, Coe RM, eds. *Nutritional intervention in the aging process.* New York: Springer–Verlag, 1984:24–47.
16. Golay A, Schutz Y, Broquet C, *et al.* Decreased thermogenic response to an oral glucose load in older subjects. *J Am Geriatr Soc* 1986;31:144–8.
17. Fukagawa NK, Bandini LG, Lim PH, Young JB. Effect of age on resting and post-prandial energy expenditure in man [Abstract]. *FASEB J* 1989;3:A934.
18. Poehlman ET, Horton ES. Regulation of energy expenditure in aging humans. *Annu Rev Nutr* 1990;10:255–75.
19. Shephard RJ. Physical training for the elderly. *Clin Sports Med* 1986;5:515–33.
20. Fiatarone MA, Evans WJ. Exercise in the oldest old. *Topics Geriatr Rehabil* 1990;5:63–77.
21. Hagberg JM. Effect of training on the decline of VO$_2$max with aging. *Fed Proc* 1987;46:1830–3.
22. Rothwell NJ, Stock MJ. Influence of noradrenaline on blood flow to brown adipose tissue in rats exhibiting diet-induced thermogenesis. *Pflugers Arch* 1981;389:237–42.
23. Robert SB, Young VR, Fuss P, *et al.* Energy expenditure and subsequent nutrient intakes in overfed young men. *Am J Physiol* 1990;259:R461–9.
24. Rudman D, Feller AG. Protein-calorie undernutrition in the nursing home. *J Am Geriatr Soc* 1989;37:173–83.
25. Meites J. Aging: hypothalamic catecholamines, neuroendocrine-immune interactions, and dietary restriction. *Proc Soc Exp Biol Med* 1990;195:304–11.
26. Pfeifer MA, Wenberg CR, Cook D, Best JD, Reeman A, Halter JB. Differential changes of autonomic nervous system function with age in man. *Am J Med* 1983;75:249–8.
27. Greenberg LH. Regulation of brain adrenergic receptors during aging. *Fed Proc* 1986;45:55–9.
28. Morley JE, Gunion MW. Central regulation of feeding: the role of neuropeptides. In: Morley JE, Sternman MB, Walsh JH, eds. *Nutrition modulation of neural function.* New York: Academic Press, 1988:125–34.
29. Nemeroff CB, Widerkiv E, Bissette G, *et al.* Increased concentrations of CSF corticotropin-releasing factor-like immunoreactivity in depressed patients. *Science* 1984;226:1342–4.
30. Morley JE. Anorexia in older patients: its meaning and management. *Geriatrics* 1990;45:59–66.
31. Fischer J, Johnson MA. Low body weight and weight loss in the aged. *J Am Diet Assoc* 1990;90:1697–706.

DISCUSSION

Dr. Schiffman: The role of palatability in energy expenditure seems to be of increasing importance. Two recent studies from England (1,2) show that thermogenesis increases when more palatable food is consumed; thus, if your food tastes good you may be less likely to get fat. Could you comment on this?

Dr. Glick: These are very interesting data. Jacques Leblanc and coworkers (3,4) found that the cephalic phase of eating involves the activation of a norepinephrine- and insulin-mediated mechanism for thermogenesis in both man and animals that is independent of nutrient absorption. I think we have the start of promising research developments in this area.

Dr. Durnin: You said that a high proportion of institutionalized elderly people suffer from protein-energy malnutrition. How did you define this?

Dr. Glick: The data are from Rudman Feller and are composite, representing the compilation of results from about 20 studies. Malnutrition was defined in two ways: first, the percentage of elderly people consuming less than their RDA; and second, indicators of poor nutrition obtained from measurements of weight for height and other anthropometric data, together with data on serum albumin and other blood indicators of nutritional status. The figures I gave referring to energy malnutrition in between 30% and 66% of institutionalized elderly were based on the physical indicators.

Dr. Durnin: None of these indicators is really satisfactory. You can have extremely well nourished people who fit all these definitions of protein-energy malnutrition. I'm not sure how much reliability we should attach to this very high percentage.

Dr. Glick: I agree that without precise standards it is difficult to produce 100% reliable estimates for the level of protein and/or energy malnutrition. However, using the same criteria the prevalence of malnutrition among healthy free-living elderly people is much lower, around 3%, so there is no doubt that there is a high prevalence of malnutrition among the institutionalized.

Dr. Mertz: People certainly eat less with increasing age, but I should like to caution against interpreting data from surveys and drawing conclusions about the adequacy of the diet. We have just reported in abstract a study done over 15 years in which we compared food intake records of 266 well trained people with food energy requirements for weight maintenance, which we determined in long-term feeding studies. We found that about 80% of our subjects underreported their usual energy intake—in other words, if we put them on their reported diet they lost weight. The average underreporting among these individuals was 25%. The intakes of essential nutrients estimated from recall surveys may therefore be substantially better than they seem.

Dr. Glick: This appears to be the consensus. However, I have focused on objective indicators rather than comparisons between reported intakes and the RDA.

Dr. Steen: I think there may be a selective underreporting of different components of the diet. For instance, when we compare urinary nitrogen excretion with dietary history data on protein intake, the correlation is surprisingly good. On the other hand, we have suspicions that there is underreporting of fat and sugar. I think we can rely on the dietary history of protein intake, however.

Dr. Hallfrisch: I have a comment about "successful aging." Normal or average aging is not necessarily particularly healthy aging. The "normal" aging person may have one or more chronic diseases and may be taking several long-term prescriptions. However, there are people who age without developing chronic diseases and without having to take drugs, and these are the successful agers. We did a longitudinal study of successful agers in which we compared men who exercised until late life with those who were sedentary but healthy and not overweight. Not only do the exercisers consume more energy, but they eat a diet of different composition. I thought this was because they were more health conscious until I heard a report of Judith Stern (5) in which she described exercising and nonexercising rats given a choice of carbohydrate, protein, and fat. The exercising rats ate more carbohydrate and the sedentary rats more fat.

Dr. Glick: I pointed out the importance of having a clear picture of changes in adiposity with advancing age. In Dr. Steen's longitudinal study, published in 1988, we see a trend to decreasing fatness in the elderly that does not reach a statistical significance. I should like to ask Dr. Steen whether his data now, after three additional years of observations, show a statistically significant decline in body fat content in older people, with advancing age.

Dr. Steen: There is a numerical trend to decreasing body fat in late age but it does not reach statistical significance. However, the proportion of the energy intake taken as fat is significantly lower in our subjects than in the Swedish population as a whole.

Dr. Nestel: Are these elderly people more health conscious? Elderly people tend to be more interested in survival than younger persons, so maybe there is a deliberate change in fat intake in a direction they think is beneficial.

Dr. Steen: We have asked this question. The answer is nearly equally divided between those who say they have reduced their fat intake for health reasons and those who say they no longer like taking much fat since it makes them feel sated.

Dr. Hallfrisch: In our data on 105 men, examining longitudinal changes in their diet over 25 years, we have shown a decline in fat intake from 42% of diet energy to 35%. Most of this decline was a secular trend seen between the 1960s and the 1980s and shared by the whole population; however, there was also a smaller, but significant, age effect such that older men ate less fat during all three decades.

REFERENCES

1. Henry CJK, Emery B. Effect of spiced food on metabolic rate: human nutrition. *Clin Nutr* 1986;40C:165–8.
2. Kimura S, Lee C. Effect of capsaicin on body fat deposition. In: Bray GA, ed. *Diet and obesity*. Basel: Japan Sci Soc Press S. Karger, 1988;219–27.
3. Diamond P, LeBlanc J. Hormonal control of postprandial thermogenesis in dogs. *Am J Physiol* 1987;253:E521–9.
4. LeBlanc J, Cabanac M. Cephalic postprandial thermogenesis in human subjects. *Physiol Behav* 1989;46:479–82.
5. Herrardo-Gettens T, Miller GD, Horwitz BA, *et al.* Exercise decreases fat selection in female rats during weight cycling. *Am J Physiol* 1991;260:R518–24.

Nutrition of the Elderly, edited by H. Munro, and
G. Schlierf, Nestlé Nutrition Workshop Series, Vol. 29,
Nestec Ltd., Vevey/Raven Press, Ltd., New York © 1992.

Protein Requirements of the Elderly

David Kritchevsky

The Wistar Institute, Philadelphia, Pennsylvania 19104, USA

Of all the chemical constituents of the organism, the ones with the widest variety
of functions are the proteins, which range from structural components to enzymes.
The proteins of animals and plants are made from the same array of about 20 amino
acids. These are all α amino acids that may have a polar, ionic side chain (PI), a
polar, non-ionic side chain (PN), or a nonpolar side chain (N), which may be aliphatic
or aromatic in nature. Table 1 lists the essential and nonessential amino acids and
indicates the polarity of the side chain.

Proteins and other amino acid–containing body constituents are being synthesized
and degraded continuously. The level of daily protein turnover is greater than can
be accounted for by ingestion, indicating that amino acids are being reused with
regularity if not total efficiency. A finite amount of nitrogenous products are excreted
and lost in sweat, sloughed skin, nails, and so forth and the amino acids thus lost
to the body's metabolic economy need constantly to be replaced.

Not all protein is digested and absorbed to the same extent. Undigested protein
and some metabolic detritus appear in the feces. The absorbed amino acids enter

TABLE 1. *The amino acids*

Essential		Nonessential	
Histidine	(PI)	Alanine	(N)
Isoleucine	(N)	Arginine	(PI)
Leucine	(N)	Asparagine	(PN)
Lysine	(PI)	Aspartic acid	(PI)
Methionine	(N)	Cysteine	(PI)
Phenylalanine	(N)	Glutamic acid	(PI)
Threonine	(PN)	Glutamine	(PN)
Tryptophan	(N)	Glycine	(N)
Valine	(N)	Hydroxyproline	(N)
		Proline	(PN)
		Serine	(PN)
		Tyrosine	(PI)

PI, polar, ionic side chain; PN, polar, non-ionic side
chain; N, neutral side chain.

the metabolic amino acid pool where they may go toward synthesis of structural or other indispensable proteins; they may be used toward maintenance of pools of cellular and circulating proteins; or they may be metabolized to CO_2 and urea. Except for those amino acids that are destined for excretion, there is an equilibrium between the amino acid pool derived from the diet and the various protein pools of the organism.

Different amino acids are used to provide different end-products, and equilibrium between precursor amino acid and its particular product can be used to measure rates of utilization. The interactions among amino acids and proteins and aspects of turnover studies have been discussed recently by Young and Fukagawa (1).

Measurement of amino acid metabolism or of protein turnover generally depends on tracing the metabolic pathway(s) of isotopically labeled amino acids. The labels are usually ^{15}N or ^{13}C, although ^{14}C has been used. Generally these are administered intravenously or by gavage and the appearance of tracer in plasma or in end-products (urea, NH_3) is measured. The data are analyzed using specific mathematical models. Another approach involves measuring the dilution by body pools of an intravenously administered labeled amino acid and using the derived data to assess protein synthesis or catabolism. The assessments can be complicated by the interactions between amino acids and the known ability of one amino acid to replace the requirement for another: tyrosine can replace 50% of the requirement for phenylalanine, for example.

Protein quality will also influence amino acid metabolism because different amounts of different proteins are absorbed. Protein quality is assessed in various ways. One is protein efficiency ratio (PER), which is determined by dividing an animal's weight gain by its protein intake. Another index, biological value (BV), is defined by the equation: (nitrogen retained/nitrogen absorbed from dietary protein) × 100. Digestibility is defined as nitrogen intake minus fecal nitrogen plus fecal metabolic nitrogen divided by nitrogen intake. Finally, net protein utilization (NPU) is defined as nitrogen retained divided by nitrogen consumed. Albanese (2) has summarized these values for some common foods. Whole egg (hen's) shows a digestibility of 99%, BV of 94%, NPU of 94%, and PER of 3.92. Beef is 99% digestible but its BV, NPU, and PER values are 74%, 73%, and 3.20, respectively. In contrast, soybeans are 90% digestible, have BV and NPU values of 73% and 66% and a PER of 2.32.

PROTEIN SYNTHESIS AND TURNOVER

Young *et al.* (3) studied total body protein synthesis in term and premature infants and young and old adults. They administered ^{15}N-glycine to achieve a steady state and then determined the isotope enrichment in urinary urea. For the purposes of this discussion we need only consider the data derived from the adult subjects. The four young adults (three male, one female) were aged 20 to 23 years and the elderly groups consisted of four women aged 69 to 91 years. In the young group (body weight

71 ± 15 kg) total body protein synthesis amounted to 3.0 ± 0.2 g/kg/day or 0.11 ± 0.01 g/calorie. In the elderly women (body weight 56 ± 10 kg), total body protein synthesis was 1.9 ± 0.2 g/kg/day or 0.11 ± 0.03 g/calorie. They concluded that the efficiency of dietary nitrogen utilization was similar for the two groups and that protein needs were a function of rate of protein synthesis.

James and Lehmann (4) compared protein turnover in small groups of fit young people (age 45–51 years), fit old people (age 68–69 years), and immobile old people (age 67–93 years) (Table 2). Although there were differences among the three groups in protein turnover, synthesis, and breakdown, protein balance was not significantly different.

A number of physical, physiological, psychological, and sociological changes occur in aging subjects. Some of these, such as the loss of lean tissue mass, reduction in liver size, and loss of renal function, may be regarded as "normal" concomitants of aging. Cohn et al. (5) described age-related changes in the body composition of men. Their body weight in the second, fourth, sixth, or seventh decade of life hardly varied (80 ± 0.4 kg) and neither did nonmuscle mass (37.5 ± 0.3 kg), but muscle mass fell from 30% of body weight at 20 to 29 years to 22.5% at 70 to 79 years. In that same time interval, body fat rose from 18.8% to 30% of body weight.

Protein synthesis at age 60 years is 40% below that at 30 years and falls by another 5% and 8% at 70 and 80 years, respectively. Muscle protein breakdown is also reduced with age. Muscle protein breakdown (g/day) per kilogram of body weight is 30% lower in 70-year-old men than in 22-year-old men and 52% lower in 76-year-old women than in those who are 20 years old (6).

Overlapping the physiological changes are increases in chronic conditions associated with aging. Bidlack et al. (7) have summarized some of the increases in chronic conditions that are observed in aging. At 65 + years (compared to the national occurrence rate), arthritis is increased by 284%, hypertension by 235%, diabetes by 246%, and diseases of the urinary tract by 124%. The prevalence of digestive diseases shows a similar pattern. Compared to people who are younger than 45 years, inci-

TABLE 2. *Protein metabolism (g/kg/day) in fit young and fit or immobile old subjects*

	Group		
	Fit young	Fit old	Immobile old
Number	6	9	13
Gender	5M; 1F	6M; 3F	6M; 7F
Mean age (yrs)	47.5	76.1	81.6
Turnover	2.833 ± 0.16	2.303 ± 0.11	2.907 ± 0.17[a]
Synthesis	2.216 ± 0.12	1.703 ± 0.09	2.220 ± 0.13[a]
Breakdown	2.083 ± 0.16	1.553 ± 0.11	2.157 ± 0.17[a]
Balance	+0.150 ± 0.5	+0.150 ± 0.5	+0.106 ± 0.09[b]

After James OFW, Lehmann AB (4).
[a] $p < 0.05$.
[b] Not significant.

dence at 65+ years of ulcer is increased by 44%, constipation by 428%, gastritis by 107%, colitis and gastroenteritis by 160%, and there is a 28-fold increase in diverticular disease (8).

Other factors also impinge on nutrition. Lowenstein (9) has pointed out that nutrition of the elderly is complicated by dental problems. About two-thirds of Americans aged 75 years have lost more than half their teeth, which influences the quality as well as quantity of food intake. A rise in the threshold for taste and smell may affect eating behavior and thus influence nutritional status. Social factors such as depression and social isolation also play a role in determining nutritional quality and adequacy. Whereas nutritional requirements of the elderly for protein are logically determined in a healthy population, the values thus derived have to be modified to fit specific cases of aging-related conditions.

PROTEIN REQUIREMENTS OF ADULTS

Protein requirements of adults are determined in one of two ways. The first of these is called the factorial method and is based on measurement of losses of nitrogen (via urine, feces, skin) and then factoring in other aspects of nitrogen metabolism. The underlying principle is to measure loss of body nitrogen when the subject is ingesting an adequate, but nitrogen-free, diet. The endogenous loss of nitrogen is assumed to be the minimum nitrogen output in subjects in the healthy state. The minimum dietary protein requirement is then the amount of high quality protein needed to balance the endogenous loss.

Nitrogen loss in urine and feces is relatively easy to measure in subjects stabilized on a protein-free diet. Minor nitrogen loss (cutaneous, etc.) is more difficult to assess but has been assumed to be about 5 mg of nitrogen/kg of body weight per day in men and 3.6 mg/kg/day in women. The obligatory body losses (urine plus feces plus skin plus miscellaneous) are taken as minimum body loss and, to correct for efficiency of nitrogen utilization, the obligatory value is multiplied by a factor of 1.3. In other words, the nitrogen requirement at that point is 130% of the obligatory loss. To account for individual variation, the nitrogen requirement is multiplied again by a factor of 1.3. This figure (now 169% of the obligatory loss) is considered to be practical and represents the "safe" nitrogen allowance. In growth, pregnancy, or lactation the nitrogen requirement is increased and again multiplied by an appropriate factor. Using this method, an FAO/WHO study concluded that 0.57 g egg protein/kg ideal weight was sufficient to meet protein requirements (10).

The other method for assessing protein requirements is to measure nitrogen balance in response to graded levels of dietary protein. Both methods have been discussed in detail by Young (11) and Munro (12). Young (11) summarized studies in which the total urinary plus fecal nitrogen loss in young women, young men, and elderly women was 1.96, 3.33, and 2.13 g, respectively. When computed on the basis of body weight, the nitrogen loss in the three groups was approximately 34 ± 4 mg/kg in young women, 46 ± 6 mg/kg in young men, and 34 ± 6 mg/kg in elderly women. He also cites data (11) suggesting that the "safe practical allowance" of milk or egg protein for elderly women is 0.42 g/kg/day.

Early reviews suggested that the protein needs of elderly people did not differ markedly from those of young people, being in the range of 0.7 to 1.0 g protein/kg/day. In the past decade or so, further studies have appeared. Cheng *et al.* (13) examined nitrogen balance in young and old adults at three levels of protein intake. This protein was derived from a mixture of wheat, soy, and milk. Their subjects were eight young prisoners (age 25.5 ± 0.9 years) and seven elderly volunteers (age 66.9 ± 1.9 years) from a Chilean nursing home. Protein intake was studied in 11-day periods using diets that provided 0.4, 0.8, or 1.6 g/kg/day. Energy intake was set at 40 kcal/kg/day. At each level of protein intake, digestibility was similar in the young and old groups. At 0.4 g nitrogen/kg/day all subjects were in negative nitrogen balance to the same extent. At 0.8 g nitrogen/kg/day, five of the young men and three of the old men were in negative nitrogen balance but there were no statistical differences between the groups. At 1.6 g nitrogen/kg/day all the subjects were in positive nitrogen balance and there was no difference between the groups. The conclusion was that there were no significant differences between young and old men in protein requirement or efficiency of utilization.

Uauy *et al.* (14) studied nitrogen balance response to graded levels of egg protein in seven elderly men and seven elderly women. The average age of the men and women was 71 and 74 years, respectively. The men were fed 0.57, 0.70, or 0.85 g protein/kg/day and the women were given 0.52, 0.65, or 0.80 g protein/kg/day. The diet periods were 10 days in duration. Of the men, four were in positive nitrogen balance on the lower levels of intake and five achieved positive nitrogen balance on the highest intake. All the women were in negative nitrogen balance at the lowest level, and five remained in negative balance at the two higher intakes. The calculated protein requirement for the women was 0.83 g/kg/day or about twice that estimated earlier by the factorial method (15). Zanni *et al.* (16) used the factorial method to measure protein requirements in six elderly (68 ± 5 years) men. They arrived at a "safe" level for egg protein of 0.59 g protein/kg ideal body weight.

Gersovitz *et al.* (17) conducted a month-long metabolic nitrogen balance study on seven elderly men (75 ± 4 years) and eight elderly women (78 ± 9 years). The subjects were ambulatory but not in the best of health. The sole protein source in the diet was 0.8 g egg protein/kg/day. About half the subjects in each group were not in nitrogen balance during the last 5 days of the study. The authors concluded that 0.8 g/kg/day of egg protein is not sufficient to confer nitrogen equilibrium in subjects older than 70 years. Their results paralleled earlier ones obtained in the same laboratory (14). The recent findings are summarized in Table 3.

Energy intake declines with aging. McGandy *et al.* (18) found in one cohort of men that energy intake fell by 22% (2,700–2,100 kcal) as their age rose from 30 to 80 years. Munro (19) reported that young men in Scotland ingested between 3,000 and 4,000 kcal/day (about 12% as protein), whereas retired men subsisted on 2,050 kcal/day (14% as protein). Kishi *et al.* (20) have shown that as energy intake of adult men fell, so did their dietary protein requirement to achieve zero nitrogen balance.

TABLE 3. *Recent studies of protein requirements in the elderly*

Subjects and methods	Conclusion	Ref.
7 men, age = 66.9 ± 5.0 years. Three 11-day periods of 0.4, 0.8, or 1.6 g/kg protein (wheat–soy–milk). Energy intake 40 kcal/mg. 57% in nitrogen balance at 0.8 g/kg	0.8 g protein/kg is adequate	13
7 men (71.3 ± 6 years); 7 women (74.0 ± 6 years). Not all in optimum health. 10-day study. Egg protein fed at 0.57, 0.70, or 0.85 g/kg (men) or 0.52, 0.65, and 0.80 g/kg (women). Energy intake 32 kcal/g. At highest level 71% men, 29% women in positive balance	0.8 g protein/kg is more adequate than FAO/WHO "safe level"	14
6 men (68.2 ± 4.8 years). Factorial method. Fed ⅓–⅛ times N loss. Energy intake 32 kcal/g	FAO/WHO "safe level" (0.57 g egg protein) is adequate	16
7 men (75.3 ± 3.9 years); 7 women (78.1 ± 9.0 years). None of the subjects truly healthy. 0.8 g egg protein for 30 days. Energy intake 32 kcal/kg (men), 29 kcal/kg (women). After 30 days 4/7 of each group in positive balance	0.8 g protein/kg not adequate in the long term	17

For instance, at an intake of 40 kcal/kg the mean requirement was 0.78 g protein/kg and at 57 kcal/kg the mean protein requirement was 0.42 g protein/kg.

Munro *et al.* (21) have recently examined the adequacy of protein intake in 691 healthy, free-living men and women. They divided the study groups by age, 60 to 75 years or >75 years. The average protein intake of the group was in the range of 1.02 to 1.06 g/kg. The authors examined the levels of a variety of plasma proteins as a function of protein intake. In the men total plasma proteins declined with increasing protein intake. Among the women there were also significant reductions in plasma transferrin, ceruloplasmin, and retinol-binding protein. The reduced levels of these proteins in aging cannot be attributed to low levels of dietary protein (Table 4).

Protein provides total nitrogen as well as essential amino acids. Are these components required in the same ratio throughout life? Munro (12) has reviewed the data and has shown that in infancy 43% of total dietary nitrogen must be in the form of essential amino acids in order to support optimal growth. At 10 to 23 years only 36% of the nitrogen need be as essential amino acids and in young adults this ratio falls to 19%. The situation in the elderly has not been resolved. Tuttle *et al.* (22) suggested that the requirement of some essential amino acids might be increased in the elderly. They found specifically that the requirements for methionine plus cystine and for lysine were 46 and 30 mg/kg, respectively (23), whereas Munro (12) cites his own data, which show the requirements for those specific amino acids to be 13 and 11 mg/kg in young adults. Albanese *et al.* (24) reported that elderly women might have an increased lysine requirement. Watts *et al.* (25) found that sulfur amino acid

TABLE 4. *Protein intake and plasma constituents in elderly men and women*

	Group			
	Men		Women	
	60–75 years	>75 years	60–75 years	>75 years
Diet				
Protein (g/day)	83	74	65	64
(g/kg/Bwt)	1.06	1.05	1.02	1.06
Energy (kJ/day)	8113	7432	6283	6182
Plasma (per dl)				
Protein (g)	7.01[a]	7.03	7.00	6.86[a]
Albumin (g)	4.23	4.11	4.20	4.05
Transferrin (mg)	298	296	303[a]	292
Ceruloplasmin (mg)	32.1	34.8	26.4[a]	35.8
Urea (mg)	29.1[b]	23.3[b]	17.1	19.9
Creatinine (mg)	1.24[a]	1.35	1.01	1.11

After Munro HN, *et al.* (21).
[a] Negatively correlated with protein intake ($p \leq 0.05$).
[b] Positively correlated with protein intake ($p \leq 0.05$).

requirements in elderly black men were lower than those for younger men. All these studies were based on protein (or amino acid) intake necessary to achieve zero nitrogen balance.

CONCLUSION

The Recommended Daily Allowances publication (26) summarized estimates of essential amino acid requirements in infants, children, and adults. Requirements (minus histidine for which there are no data in children aged 2–12 years) fall from 714 mg/kg/day in infants, to 352 mg/kg/day in children under the age of 2, to 214 mg/kg/day in children aged 10 to 12, and down to 84 mg/kg/day in adults. Thus, the reduction in requirement between 3 months and adulthood is 88%. The foregoing discussion suggests that we need to learn more about essential amino acid requirements in the elderly.

A high protein intake may be detrimental in that it may increase calcium excretion (27) and may influence age-related loss of kidney function (28). However, other experiments have shown that the increased calcium excretion may only be transient (29), and one long-term study did not show any correlation between protein intake, aging, and kidney function (30).

The data that we have available at present suggest that health in aging (for subjects with no debilitating disease) can be maintained on an average daily intake of 1 g protein per kg body weight or less (23). The new recommended dietary allowance for men and women older than 51 years is 0.8 g/kg body weight, or an average of 63 g/day for men and 50 g/day for women (26).

In view of the increasing proportion of the elderly in the population, we could profit from further investigations into requirements for specific amino acids, and it might also be useful to study further the influences of protein and amino acid intakes on the metabolism of specific proteins. The classification of elderly used by Munro *et al.* (21), namely, 60 to 75 years and 76+ years, could further focus our knowledge of protein requirements.

ACKNOWLEDGMENT

Supported in part by a Research Career Award (HL 00734) from the National Institutes of Health and by funds from the Commonwealth of Pennsylvania.

REFERENCES

1. Young VR, Fukagawa NK. Amino acid interactions: a selective review. In: Boldwell CE, Erdman JW, eds. *Nutrient interactions*. New York: Marcel Dekker, 1988:27–71.
2. Albanese AA. Protein needs. In: Albanese AA, ed. *Nutrition for the elderly*. New York: Alan R Liss, 1980:35–65.
3. Young VR, Steffee WP, Pencharz PB, Winterer JC, Scrimshaw NS. Total human body protein synthesis in relation to protein requirements at various ages. *Nature* 1975;253:192–3.
4. James OFW, Lehmann AB. Protein metabolism in the elderly. *Topics Aging Res Eur* 1986;10: 25–30.
5. Cohn SH, Vartsky D, Yasumura S, *et al.* Compartmental body composition based on total-body nitrogen, potassium and calcium. *Am J Physiol* 1980;239:E524–30.
6. Uauy R, Winterer JC, Bilmazes C, *et al.* The changing pattern of whole body protein metabolism in aging humans. *J Gerontol* 1978;33:663–71.
7. Bidlack WR, Smith CH, Clemens RA, Omaye ST. Nutrition and the elderly. *Food Technol* 1986;40:81–8.
8. Young EA, Urban E. Aging, the aged and the gastrointestinal tract. In: Young EA, ed. *Nutrition, aging and health*. New York: Alan R Liss, 1986:91–131.
9. Lowenstein FW. Nutritional requirements of the elderly. In: Young EA, ed. *Nutrition, aging and health*. New York: Alan R Liss, 1986:61–89.
10. Joint FAO/WHO Expert Committee on Energy and Protein Requirements. *Energy and protein requirements*. World Health Organization Technical Report Series No 522. Geneva: World Health Organization, 1973.
11. Young VR. Protein metabolism and needs in elderly people. In: Rockstein M, Sussman MJ, eds. *Nutrition, longevity and aging*. New York: Academic Press, 1976:67–102.
12. Munro HN. Protein nutriture and requirements of the elderly. In: Munro HN, Danford DE, eds. *Nutrition, aging and the elderly*. New York: Plenum Press, 1989:153–81.
13. Cheng AHR, Gomez A, Bergan JG, Lee TC, Monckeberg F, Chichester CO. Comparative nitrogen balance study between young and aged adults using three levels of protein intake from a combination wheat-soy-milk mixture. *Am J Clin Nutr* 1978;31:12–22.
14. Uauy R, Scrimshaw NS, Young VR. Human protein requirements: nitrogen balance response to graded levels of egg protein in elderly men and women. *Am J Clin Nutr* 1978;31:779–85.
15. Scrimshaw NS, Perera WDA, Young VR. Protein requirements of man: obligatory urinary and fecal nitrogen losses in elderly women. *J Nutr* 1976;106:665–70.
16. Zanni E, Calloway DH, Zezulka AY. Protein requirements of elderly men. *J Nutr* 1979;109:513–24.
17. Gersovitz M, Motil K, Munro HM, Scrimshaw NS, Young VR. Human protein requirements: assessment of the adequacy of the current recommended dietary allowance for dietary protein in elderly men and women. *Am J Clin Nutr* 1982;35:6–14.
18. McGandy RB, Barrows CH, Spanias A, Meredith A, Stone JL, Norris AH. Nutrient intakes and energy expenditure in men of different ages. *J Gerontol* 1966;21:581–7.
19. Munro HN. An introduction to nutritional aspects of protein metabolism. In: Munro HN, Allison JB, eds. *Mammalian protein metabolism*, vol 2. New York: Academic Press, 1964:3–39.

20. Kishi K, Miyatani S, Inoue G. Requirement and utilization of egg protein by Japanese young men with marginal intakes of energy. *J Nutr* 1978;109:658–69.
21. Munro HN, McGandy RB, Hartz SC, Russell RM, Jacob RA, Otradovec CL. Protein nutriture of a group of free-living elderly. *Am J Clin Nutr* 1987;46:586–92.
22. Tuttle SG, Swendseid ME, Mulcare D, Griffith WH, Bassett SH. Study of the essential amino acid requirements of men over fifty. *Metabolism* 1957;6:564–73.
23. Tuttle SG, Bassett SH, Griffith WH, Mulcare DB, Swendseid ME. Further observations on amino acid requirements of older men II. Methionine and lysine. *Am J Clin Nutr* 1965;16:229–31.
24. Albanese AA, Higgens RA, Orto LA, Zwattoro DN. Protein and amino acid needs in the aged in health and convalescence. *Geriatrics* 1957;12:443–52.
25. Watts JH, Mann AN, Bradley L, Thompson DJ. Nitrogen balances of men over 65 fed the FAO and milk patterns of essential amino acids. *J Gerontol* 1964;19:370–4.
26. Food and Nutrition Board. Subcommittee on the tenth edition of the RDA "Recommended Dietary Allowances." Washington, DC: National Academy of Sciences, 1989:52–77.
27. Anand CR, Linksweiler HM. Effect of protein intake on calcium balance of young men given 500 mg calcium daily. *J Nutr* 1974;104:695–700.
28. Brenner BM, Meyer TW, Hostetter TH. Dietary protein and the progressive nature of kidney disease: the role of hemodynamically mediated glomerular injury in the pathogenesis of progressive glomerular sclerosis in aging, renal ablation and intrinsic renal disease. *N Engl J Med* 1982;307:652–9.
29. Spencer H, Kramer L, Osis D, Norris C. Effect of a high protein (meat) intake on calcium metabolism in man. *Am J Clin Nutr* 1978;36:2167–80.
30. Tobin J. Nutrition and organ function in a cohort of aging men. In: Hutchinson ML, Munro HM, eds. *Nutrition and aging.* New York: Academic Press, 1986:23–34.

DISCUSSION

Dr. Munro: It is important to recognize that nitrogen balance is affected to a major extent by the amount of energy in the diet. You can easily turn a negative balance into a positive one and vice versa by altering the energy intake.

Dr. Rush: Dr. Meredith may wish to comment on data that suggest that a protein intake of 0.6 or even 0.8 g/kg is inadequate for older individuals who exercise regularly. Also, although I don't find the data compelling, it is worth recalling that Colin Campbell believes that the high protein levels of Western diets may be more harmful for health than their high fat content. There is a considerable literature on protein toxicity from fetal life through old age.

Dr. Meredith: Using nitrogen balances, we have found that active men in late middle age do indeed have a higher nitrogen requirement than sedentary individuals—about 0.95 g/kg daily. Energy intakes in these men were very large compared with sedentary subjects. However, if protein is considered as a fraction of the energy intake, the protein requirement was actually lower than in sedentary subjects.

Dr. Glick: Is Dr. Meredith suggesting that the increased requirement for protein in active people is associated with their higher level of activity? Could it not be accounted for simply by their having a greater muscle mass?

Dr. Meredith: The people we were studying were runners or cyclists. Their muscle mass was not obviously different from sedentary individuals. Therefore, I don't think the size of the muscle compartment was important in explaining the differences. I favor the hypothesis that has been put forward from England that suggests that if you have a high rate of energy expenditure, protein is burned along with other fuels at a greater rate than usual.

I should like to make a further comment that is perhaps more relevant to aging. I don't think we have sufficiently examined protein and energy requirements in an extremely sedentary population. I wonder whether the relationships that Dr. Munro has described between protein intake and energy intake are changed by the combination of immobilization and old age.

Dr. Berry: When you are looking for a cheap source of protein of high biological value for elderly people on a reduced budget, is there anything to compare with eggs?

Dr. Kritchevsky: Not in my view. I think eggs are the best and cheapest source of high grade protein. If you are a fanatic about cholesterol you can use the white only, but the yolk contains a lot of phospholipid and is fairly high in monounsaturates.

Dr. Munro: It is important to emphasize that the degree of chronic illness in elderly people is relevant to their protein requirements. In a British study population, all but one of those individuals who were identified as having some clinically or biochemically recognizable form of malnutrition had chronic wasting diseases (1). I do not think it is reasonable to legislate only for the healthy. We must legislate for people who need additional energy and protein to compensate for the ravages of chronic disease.

Dr. Kritchevsky: This is more or less what I said at the end of my paper. We need to start to look at different groups of elderly people ranging from the healthy to the sick. I think it is a grave error that the RDAs stop at 51 + years of age.

Dr. Durnin: What sort of difference would it make to the true protein requirements for people with wasting diseases? Would you add 0.2 g/kg?

Dr. Munro: I imagine that is the order of magnitude that would be required.

Dr. Nestel: What is known about protein requirements in less developed parts of the world? There are data from New Guinea collected in the early 1970s that suggested that the protein intake was less than half the FAO recommended value, yet the subjects were muscular fit old people.

Dr. Munro: Those studies have been criticized because of the method of nitrogen collection and other methodological problems.

Dr. Nestel: It is true that the measurements of nitrogen excretion were suboptimal, but the diet was very simple and readily measurable and nearly all nutritionists working in the area said that about 90% of the diet was carbohydrate. This doesn't leave much for fat and protein, however one calculates it.

Dr. Berry: What is considered to be the best biochemical index or test for detecting an inadequate protein intake?

Dr. Munro: Nitrogen balance has been the standard since about 1840, but it is not an easy technique to apply with the necessary precision. The somatomedin factors (insulin-like growth factors, or IGFs) might be helpful, although it may simply reflect the rate of protein turnover. We don't yet know whether it is really sensitive to the balance of protein, represented by the difference between intake and requirement.

Dr. Nestel: Data from my institution show that in the early years of life infection and nitrogen loss are associated with low plasma IGF concentrations and the IGF levels increase as the children recover from illness and nitrogen balance becomes positive.

Dr. Heseker: We have heard a lot about the decrease in lean body mass with age. To what degree can elderly people diminish this decrease by physical exertion?

Dr. Meredith: The decrease in lean mass with age does not seem to be affected by activity levels. Men who have been athletes all their lives remain extremely fit but still sustain loss of lean mass. However, we need more data on different types of exercise that might maintain or increase lean mass in the elderly.

REFERENCE

1. Department of Health and Social Security. *A nutrition survey of the elderly.* Reports on health and social subjects no 16. London: Department of Health and Social Services. HMSO, 1979.

Nutrition of the Elderly, edited by H. Munro, and
G. Schlierf, Nestlé Nutrition Workshop Series, Vol. 29,
Nestec Ltd., Vevey/Raven Press, Ltd., New York © 1992.

Dietary Fat for the Elderly: What Are the Issues?

Paul J. Nestel

CSIRO Division of Human Nutrition, The Flinders University of South Australia, Adelaide SA 5000, Australia

Several major chronic diseases that afflict the elderly are in part related to excess dietary fat. This needs to be balanced against the nutritive value of fat and the tendency for elderly people to eat less fat by choice. Recommendations to the elderly on how much fat they should eat are therefore complex. What type of fat to eat is simpler.

Food lipids have many nutritional and biological functions as well as organoleptic properties. In the past, people have selected fat-containing foods for the flavor and texture and not the nutritive value, which fat imparts. Fats are a major source of energy, the source of the fat-soluble vitamins (A, D, E, and K) that have numerous regulatory effects, and the source of two essential fatty acids, linoleic and α-linolenic acids. The n-6 and n-3 fatty acids generate the potent eicosanoids, cellular signal transduction is influenced by inositol phosphatides, and cholesterol is the precursor of bile acids and of steroid hormones. The question is whether a significant reduction in dietary fats would jeopardize the adequate intake of these fat-dependent nutrients.

FOOD CONSUMPTION PATTERNS

Elderly people tend to eat less (1) partly in response to reduced physical activity, and partly for social and health reasons. Appetite and smell decline, while loneliness, depression, and inability to buy and prepare food reduce the incentive to eat adequately. Eating less fat is common and along with this goes the possibility of eating fewer fat-soluble vitamins. This possibility has been investigated with the general finding that in healthy elderly people there is little evidence for deficiency in vitamins A, D, and E (1). Nevertheless, the average consumption of vitamin D and of calcium is marginal and below recommended daily intakes in up to one-quarter of the older Australian population (2).

Dr. Katrine Baghurst in the Division of Human Nutrition, CSIRO, Adelaide, has unpublished data on the profile of fat consumption in older Australians. Total fat consumption is only a little below the national average for adults (33% vs. 35% of

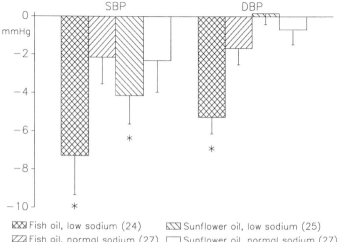

FIG. 1. Falls in systolic blood pressure (SBP) and in diastolic blood pressure (DBP) after 6 weeks of four dietary interventions. The two cross-over periods are: **(i)** a low sodium intake together with either fish oil or sunflower oil; **(ii)** a normal sodium intake together with either fish oil or sunflower oil. (Number of subjects in parentheses.)

dietary energy). The proportions derived from saturates, monounsaturates, and polyunsaturates also resemble the national profile. Dietary cholesterol consumption is below average (230 mg for women and 290 mg for men), reflecting recent dietary changes in the direction of less animal fat (Fig. 1). The calculated intakes of vitamins A and E are adequate. This contrasts with McGandy's findings in elderly people in Boston (3), who eat substantially reduced amounts of fat and calcium.

OVERWEIGHT

Lean body mass decreases and fat mass increases with aging. This probably reflects lower physical activity and possibly reduced resting metabolic rate (4). These factors predispose to obesity and raise questions about the role of total fat intake in the process of becoming fat and whether obesity is an important health risk in older people.

A recent prospective survey of men and women aged 55 to 74 years at entry found no additional risk for women attributable to overweight, provided there was no other clinical condition related to fatness (5). Among men who were frankly obese (>30 kg/m^2), the relative risk was slightly increased over the 8.7 years of follow-up (1.1–1.2). However, low body weight (<22 kg/m^2) was associated with substantial increases in mortality and morbidity that were independent of smoking. This important finding, observed in other prospective studies, raises the question whether restricting dietary fat is advisable for older people who are otherwise free of disorders that are adversely influenced by fat.

LIPID METABOLISM AND CORONARY HEART DISEASE

The major public health indication to change the nature of dietary fatty acids relates to lowering plasma cholesterol levels and consequently reducing coronary heart disease. Until recently, this was taken to be pertinent only to younger adults but this view is now being recast to include older people as well.

The first question to ask is whether cholesterol metabolism changes with aging, making a rise in the plasma cholesterol concentration inevitable. It should be noted that in some non-Western societies this rise does not occur (6). It has been postulated that the activity of the low-density lipoprotein (LDL) receptor declines with age but in the absence of a reliable assay in a readily available human tissue, we have no answer. It seems likely, though, that diminished LDL removal rather than overproduction is the cause of the age-related cholesterol rise.

The importance of this is that the plasma cholesterol, or more properly the LDL cholesterol concentration, remains an independent risk factor into old age. The Honolulu Heart Study showed this to be the case in men older than 65 years (7); this is confirmed in the most recent analysis of the Framingham cohort (8).

Equally, elevated high-density lipoprotein (HDL) cholesterol confers protection in older as well as in younger people (9). Interestingly, octogenarians in the Framingham study were exceedingly unlikely to have reduced HDL cholesterol levels (10). A cross-sectional survey of 1280 80-year-old men in Sweden found them to have a moderately low average plasma cholesterol concentration, suggesting selective mortality (11). Nevertheless, even at such an old age raised LDL cholesterol levels predicted cardiovascular disease. The implications are that national strategies to counter coronary disease by reducing the average cholesterol level also apply to the elderly.

Raised plasma triglyceride levels are now also generally recognized as increasing cardiovascular risk, more so in women than in men (12). This is particularly true for aortofemoral atherosclerosis and when hypertriglyceridemia occurs as part of a lipoprotein phenotype which includes low HDL and/or raised LDL cholesterol (12). The rise in plasma triglyceride that accompanies aging therefore deserves remedial action.

Apart from increased fat mass, another recognized reason for the rising triglyceride concentration is reduced removal. The key control enzyme, lipoprotein lipase, falls with aging (13) and this is reflected in the prolongation of lipemia after a fat meal (14). If LDL receptor activity declines with aging, then the clearance of very low density lipoprotein (VLDL) remnants, derived from endogenous synthesis of triglyceride, will also be impaired. This in turn will aggravate the removal of chylomicron remnants, since the two products of triglyceride catabolism compete for common degradation sites.

The strategy to manage hyperlipidemia is identical to that in the general population and includes a reduction in saturated fatty acid and substitution by a mix of polyunsaturated and monounsaturated fatty acids and complex carbohydrates.

POLYUNSATURATED FATTY ACIDS AND EICOSANOIDS

It has been suggested that polyunsaturated fatty acids, mainly linoleic acid, may pose special problems, particularly in the elderly. Quite clearly, there are benefits in terms of cholesterol reduction. The n-3 polyunsaturated fatty acids (α-linolenic, eicosapentaenoic or EPA, and docosahexaenoic or DHA) also have advantages and disadvantages. The correct balance of these two classes of fatty acids is a major challenge for nutritionists and food manufacturers. These points are discussed later.

The most important metabolites of polyunsaturated fatty acids are the eicosanoids. The nature of eicosanoids is profoundly affected by the type of dietary fatty acids. Since these products influence cardiovascular functions, thrombosis, inflammation, immunity, and probably tumor promotion, the importance of optimizing dietary fatty acids is particularly relevant in the elderly. Several of the key cellular events in atherogenesis are also affected by eicosanoids.

Eicosanoids comprise prostanoids (prostaglandins and thromboxanes) and leukotrienes. Depending on the number of double bonds, these metabolites are classified as belonging to the 1-, 2-, or 3-series. The 2-series of prostanoids (PGI_2 and TXA_2) is derived from linoleic acid and is the most potent. The 3-series, derived from EPA and DHA, is much less potent and indeed reduces the activity of the 2-series. It is therefore clear that the ratio of the 2- and 3-series and hence of their precursors, the n-6 and n-3 fatty acids, will determine key biological functions and influence many of the diseases of aging. For instance, immune responses are enhanced when tissue linoleate levels fall. Most of the evidence derives from experimental animals in which high intakes of linoleic acid (and low intakes of n-3 fatty acids) suppress immunological competence and hence interfere with the control of tumor growth.

Experimental atherogenesis is also inhibited by n-3 fatty acids derived from fish oils (15). This results from suppression of several processes: attraction of lipid-laden circulating monocytes to the arterial endothelium, adhesion of those cells to endothelium, aggregation of platelets, and production of local growth factors.

The role of the 1-series of prostanoids, especially PGI_1, is controversial. The initial step in the conversion of linoleic acid to arachidonic acid (the immediate precursor of the eicosanoids) is the insertion of a third double bond to produce γ-linolenic acid (still an n-6 fatty acid). This step is mediated by the enzyme Δ6-desaturase. It has been claimed that this enzyme declines with age (16) and that this relative deficiency gives rise to several chronic disorders that are common in the elderly. γ-Linolenic acid gives rise to dihomo-γ-linolenic acid, which can give rise to PGI_1 and/or be further desaturated to arachidonic acid. PGI_1 is claimed to have functions that oppose PGI_2. Further linoleic acid can competitively inhibit 6-desaturase activity (17).

Recently Abraham *et al.* (18) have reported low adipose levels of dihomo-γ-linolenic acid in men with coronary heart disease. Based on these observations and assumptions, Horrobin and Manku (19) have recommended increased consumption of γ-linolenic-acid–rich oils (black currant, evening primrose). The controversy can only be clarified through experiments in which purified γ-linolenic or dihomo-γ-linolenic acids are eaten.

Polyunsaturated fatty acids appear to influence the outcome of another common cause of death in the elderly: sudden cardiac arrest. Further, the extent of myocardial infarction, and the consequences of prolonged ischemia such as myocardial stunning, may also be favorably limited by fish n-3 fatty acids.

Apart from the well known low incidence of cardiac deaths in populations with high fish consumption, there is also evidence that the EPA content of blood platelets is inversely related to clinical coronary heart disease (20). Men who had died suddenly from cardiac causes were found to have reduced DHA:arachidonic acid ratios in cardiac phospholipids (21). Finally, the single intervention study with fish and fish oils in men after myocardial infarction suggested reduction in sudden cardiac deaths (22).

N-3 fatty acids may therefore protect against tachyarrhythmias and minimize infarction. Supporting evidence of this has been obtained in experimental animal studies. Animals that were fed fish oil and subsequently subjected to myocardial ischemia have shown less damage to muscle (23), and low mortality from arrhythmias (24). Some of the protective mechanisms include diminished oxygen-related free radicals, prevention of abnormal calcium fluxes, leukocyte infiltration of myocardium, and lessened eicosanoid production (25).

Importantly, McLennan *et al.* (24) have shown that aging predisposes the rat heart to ventricular arrhythmia and that this is preventable by prefeeding with fish oil.

We have found that marine n-3 fatty acids lower blood pressure potently in elderly people (26). This was seen in the context of a moderate reduction of salt intake, probably because the elderly tend to be salt-sensitive. In 105 men and women aged 60 to 80 years, a combination of 4.2 g n-3 fatty acid (2.5 g EPA + 1.7 g DHA) plus an 80-mmol reduction in NaCl, lowered systolic and diastolic pressure by 7.3 and 5.3 mmHg, respectively. The study was carried out in a double-blind cross-over design, using a normal NaCl intake or sunflower oil for comparison (Fig. 1). We believe that EPA and DHA negate the hormonal and circulatory compensating mechanisms through which volume and pressure are normally maintained during salt deprivation.

It is nevertheless important that some of the potential hazards of excessive fish n-3 fatty acids are recognized, among which the increased tendency to bleed may become more easily manifest in elderly people. The suppression of inflammatory responses that may be beneficial in some disease states may be undesirable at other times.

N-3 fatty acids may adversely affect another common disorder of the elderly: glucose intolerance, reflecting resistance of tissues to the action of insulin. It may lead to frank diabetes mellitus and to hyperlipidemia [mostly hypertriglyceridemia, low HDL, and raised apolipoprotein B (15)]. This may be aggravated by the use of n-3 fatty acids because insulin secretion may be inhibited (27).

Another postulated adverse consequence of eating polyunsaturated fatty acids is the generation of oxidized lipoproteins. The concern comes from the heightened atherogenicity of oxidized LDL; whether aging predisposes to oxidation is uncertain. A preliminary report suggests that this may be so at least for elderly women taking fish oil (28). Lipid peroxides rose in the plasma to higher levels in the older than in the younger women, but this could not be related to lesser availability of vitamin E (a natural antioxidant).

It has frequently been suggested that linoleic acid may promote cancer. Whereas the association between total fat consumption and several human cancers is supported in epidemiological surveys, there is no clear link with fatty acid type. Although experimental tumors in animals can be promoted by high linoleate diets, there is little to suggest that this is so in humans (29). Even the often quoted finding of increased colon cancer among elderly men in the Los Angeles diet trial was subsequently overturned by the original authors (30). Careful scrutiny of similar trials showed no evidence for a dietary linoleic acid–cancer link (29). At the same time, the possibility that a high n-3 fatty acid intake may be protective must be considered. A preliminary report from the Multi Risk Factor Intervention Trial (MRFIT) has reported an inverse relationship between consumption of either plant or fish n-3 fatty acids and cancer (31).

ESSENTIAL FATTY ACIDS

The requirements for linoleic acid and for α-linolenic acid are relatively small given the high intakes of both in Western societies. There is no evidence that the need for these two essential fatty acids changes with aging. The average consumption of linoleic acid in Western diets ranges between 4% and nearly 10% of daily energy, far in excess of the 1% to 2% needed. The amount of α-linolenic acid (n-3) that gives rise to EPA and DHA is less than 0.5% of total energy and is present in abundance in plants. It is now generally accepted to be an essential fatty acid also.

RECOMMENDATIONS

1. The elderly can participate in the general population strategy for a modest reduction in fat consumption. The objective is to reduce the risk of coronary heart disease by lowering plasma cholesterol, which remains a risk in older people. Cancer risk may also become less.
2. However, elderly people should not reduce fat intake markedly. They tend to eat less by choice so that further restriction of fat may lead to nutritional deficiency.
3. Weight reduction through fat restriction is not justified in the absence of obesity-related risk factors. Abnormally low body weight carries greater mortality in the elderly than overweight.
4. The nature of dietary fatty acids should resemble that advised for the population as a whole: less saturated fat and more unsaturated fat. However, there is a strong case for reducing the n-6:n-3 ratio, that is, increasing the proportions of n-3 fatty acids from plants and fish. Excess linoleic acid may interfere with immunological processes and aggravate inflammatory responses, atherogenicity, thrombosis, and possibly tumor formation, disorders to which the elderly are prone.

5. Lifestyle measures such as physical activity should be encouraged to stimulate normal eating and reduce the risk of nutrient inadequacy. However, it is most unlikely that the elderly are at risk from essential fatty acid deficiency.

REFERENCES

1. Munro HN, Suter PM, Russell RM. Nutritional requirements of the elderly. *Annu Rev Nutr* 1987;7: 23–49.
2. Department of Community Services & Health. *National dietary survey of adults, 1983.* Canberra: Australian Government Publishing Service, 1987.
3. McGandy RB, Russell RM, Hartz SC, *et al.* Nutritional status survey of healthy non-institutionalized elderly: energy and nutrient intakes from three-day diet records and nutrient supplements. *Nutr Res* 1986;6:785–98.
4. Poehlman ET, McAuliffe TL, Van Houten DR, Danforth E. Influence of age and endurance training on metabolic rate and hormones in healthy men. *Am J Physiol* 1990;259:E66–72.
5. Tayback M, Kumanyika S, Chee E. Body weight as a risk factor in the elderly. *Arch Intern Med* 1990;150:1065–72.
6. Wyatt GB, Griew AR, Martin FIR, Campbell DG. Plasma cholesterol, triglyceride and uric acid in urban and rural communities in Papua New Guinea. *Aust NZ J Med* 1980;10:491–5.
7. Benfante R, Reed D. Is elevated serum cholesterol level a risk factor for coronary heart disease in the elderly? *JAMA* 1990;263:393–6.
8. Castelli WP, Garrison RJ, Wilson PW, Abbott RD, Kalousdian S, Kannel WB. Incidence of coronary heart disease and lipoprotein cholesterol levels. The Framingham Study. *JAMA* 1986;256:2835–8.
9. Gordon T, Kannel WB, Castelli WP, *et al.* Lipoproteins, cardiovascular disease and death. The Framingham Study. *Arch Intern Med* 1981;141:1128–31.
10. Schaefer EJ, Moussa PB, Wilson PWF, McGee D, Dallal G, Castelli WP. Plasma lipoproteins in healthy octogenarians: lack of reduced high density lipoprotein cholesterol levels: results from the Framingham Heart Study. *Metabolism* 1989;38:293–6.
11. Stavenow L, Elmst AHL S, Jerntorp P, *et al.* Eighty-year old men without cardiovascular disease in the community of Malmo. Part I. Social and medical factors, with special reference to the lipoprotein pattern. *J Intern Med* 1990;228:9–15.
12. Nestel PJ. New lipoprotein profiles and coronary heart disease. *Circulation* 1990;82:649–51.
13. Huttunen JK, Ehnholm C, Kekki M, Nikkila EA. Post-heparin plasma lipoprotein lipase and hepatic lipase in normal subjects and in patients with hypertriglyceridemia: correlations to sex, age and various parameters of triglyceride metabolism. *J Sci Mol Med* 1976;50:249–60.
14. Krasinski SD, Cohn JS, Schaefer EJ, Russell RM. Postprandial plasma retinyl ester response is greater in older subjects compared with younger subjects. *J Clin Invest* 1990;85:883–92.
15. Nestel PJ. Effects of n-3 fatty acids on lipid metabolism. *Annu Rev Nutr* 1990;10:149–67.
16. Brenner RR. Nutritional and hormonal factors influencing desaturation of essential fatty acids. *Prog Lipid Res* 1981;20:41–7.
17. Kinsella JE. Food lipids and fatty acids: importance in food quality, nutrition, and health. *Food Technol* 1988;42:124–45.
18. Abraham RD, Riemersma RA, Elton RA, Macintyre C, Oliver MF. Effects of safflower oil and evening primrose oil in men with a low dihomo-gamma-linolenic level. *Atherosclerosis* 1990;81:199–208.
19. Horrobin DF, Manku MS. How do polyunsaturated fatty acids lower plasma cholesterol levels? *Lipids* 1983;18:558–62.
20. Wood DA, Riemersma RA, Butler S, *et al.* Linoleic and eicosapentaenoic acids in adipose tissues and platelets and risk of coronary heart disease. *Lancet* 1987;i:177–83.
21. Gudbjarnason S. Dynamics of n-3 and n-6 fatty acids in phospholipids of heart muscle. *J Intern Med* 1989;225:117–28.
22. Burr ML, Fehily AM, Gilbert JF, *et al.* Effects of changes in fat, fish and fibre intakes on death and myocardial reinfarction: diet and reinfarction trial (DART). *Lancet* 1989;ii:757–61.
23. Culp BR, Lands WEM, Luccesi BR, *et al.* The effect of dietary supplementation of fish oil on experimental myocardial infarction. *Prostaglandins* 1980;20:1021–31.
24. McLennan PL, Abeywardena MY, Charnock JS. The influence of age and dietary fat in an animal model of sudden cardiac death. *Aust NZ J Med* 1989;19:1–5.

25. Nestel PJ. Review: fish oil and cardiac function. *World Rev Nutr Diet* 1990;66:268–77.
26. Cobiac L, Nestel PJ, Wing LMH, Howe PRC. The effects of dietary sodium restriction and fish oil supplements on blood pressure in the elderly. *Clin Exp Pharm Physiol* 1991;18:265–8.
27. Vessby B. Effects of ω3 fatty acids on glucose and lipid metabolism in non-insulin-dependent diabetes mellitus. *World Rev Nutr Diet* 1991;66:407–16.
28. Meydani M, Natiello F, Free N, Wood M, Blumberg J, Gorbach SL. Plasma vitamin E and lipid peroxide status after long-term fish oil supplementation in young and older women. *FASEB J* 1990;4:A1157.
29. Ederer F, Leren P, Turpeinen O, Frandt ID. Cancer among men on cholesterol-lowering diets. Experience from five clinical trials. *Lancet* 1971;i:203–5.
30. Heyden S. Polyunsaturated fatty acids and colon cancer. *Nutr Med* 1974;17:321–6.
31. Dolacek TA, Grandits G. Dietary polyunsaturated fatty acids and mortality in the Multiple Risk Factor Intervention Trial (MRFIT). *World Rev Nutr Diet* 1991;66:205–16.

DISCUSSION

Dr. Kritchevsky: Could you summarize Dolachek's findings on n-3 fatty acids in the MRFIT study?

Dr. Nestel: The findings relate to 18,000 people in the MRFIT study who took part in nutrition surveys and intervention studies (1). There was a twofold difference in mortality from coronary heart disease (CHD) and cancer in favor of n-3 fatty acids between the lowest and the highest n-3 intake quintiles. When other risks such as high blood pressure, unfavorable plasma lipids, and smoking were taken into account, a greater benefit from n-3 fatty acids was shown.

Dr. Meredith: Canola oil is becoming very popular. Do you have any reservations about older people increasing their intake of this type of oil?

Dr. Nestel: If you asked me what was the optimal fatty acid mix in the diet, I should say it closely resembles canola oil, which has 9% saturated fatty acids, 50% oleic acid, and a good ratio of linoleic to linolenic acids. I do not believe there is a case for restricting fat in the elderly unless there is a specific reason to do so. Of all the oils, I think canola oil may be the most desirable.

Dr. Rush: Would you comment on the potential entry into the food supply of sucrose polyester and what it might do to vitamin requirements?

Dr. Nestel: For the population as a whole, I don't have any major reservations, but in elderly people taking a restricted energy intake, and hence a restricted fat intake, a further reduction in available fat solubility for fat-associated nutrients would be compromised by sucrose polyester.

Dr. Stern: I feel that elderly people should be advised to lower their fat intake, but the reason should be to limit empty calories and thus help maintain their intake of essential nutrients, rather than, for example, to lower their total blood cholesterol. What are your views on this?

Dr. Nestel: I am not so concerned about the quantity of fat but rather about the fatty acid mix within the dietary fat. I have looked at this very narrowly from the point of view of healthy individuals with no relevant risk factors. Nevertheless, I think one should be considering what a high fat diet might be doing to glucose intolerance, which is obviously a common condition in the elderly, or what its role might be in cancer of the colon. These matters are still under review. My feeling at present is that there is no urgency for the elderly to lower their fat intake but that we should be thinking about altering the nature of the fatty acids.

Dr. Kritchevsky: Could you comment on triglycerides as a possible risk factor?

Dr. Nestel: Triglycerides are making a bit of a comeback. One reason for this may be the recognition that hypertriglyceridemia alone is not really a very common cause of CHD but that the hypertriglyceridemia that causes coronary heart disease is usually the high triglyceride, low HDL syndrome, or combined hyperlipoproteinemia in which LDLs are raised also. One problem in the past was a failure to recognize the large biological and diurnal fluctuations in triglyceride levels, so that when triglycerides were measured on one occasion only, they couldn't possibly be as good an index as the HDL cholesterol, which varies relatively little from day to day.

Dr. Berry: I'm interested in your statement that the strategy for hyperlipidemia in the elderly should be the same as for younger age groups. I find it hard to believe that someone with hypercholesterolemia at the age of 70 has the same risk as someone at the age of 30. Elderly people with hypercholesterolemia probably have as yet unknown protective factors. If you feel an intervention is essential, then surely it would be best to try to raise HDL by exercise and to try to modify the habitual diet by manipulating the polyunsaturated/saturated (PS) ratio, which is anyway rather high in your population.

Dr. Nestel: Aortic atherosclerosis and carotid atherosclerosis are disorders that occur a decade later than coronary heart disease. Aortic atherosclerosis in particular is strongly correlated with hypertriglyceridemia. I believe the nutritional strategies I have outlined are not harmful and may be beneficial.

REFERENCE

1. Dolacek TA, Grandits G. Dietary polyunsaturated fatty acids and mortality in the Multiple Risk Factor intervention trial (MRFIT). Health effects of omega 3 polyunsaturated fatty acids in seafoods. *World Rev Nutr Diet* 1991;66:205–16.

Nutrition of the Elderly, edited by H. Munro, and
G. Schlierf, Nestlé Nutrition Workshop Series, Vol. 29,
Nestec Ltd., Vevey/Raven Press, Ltd., New York © 1992.

Vitamin Requirements of the Elderly

Helmut Heseker and Werner Kübler

Institute of Nutrition, Justus-Liebig-University, D-6300 Giessen, Germany

Up to now nutritionists have not reached an agreement on the absolute daily requirement and its range for all vitamins. The reason for these scientific differences
in opinion is largely attributable on the one hand to methodological or technical
problems and on the other hand to terminological difficulties (1). Disagreement like-
wise exists as to whether the classic definitions of the minimum requirement[a] should
remain or whether it would be more practical to identify the requirement as the intake
necessary to maintain a defined level (higher than at present) of vitamin stores.
Results from epidemiological studies support this concept in relation to the vitamins
with antioxidative properties, such as ascorbic acid, tocopherol, and β-carotene.

Nutrient intakes considered adequate for the elderly (3,4) are often based on extrapolation from the better defined requirements of younger adults, partly by taking
the changed energy needs into consideration. Fortunately, the question about specific needs for vitamins in the elderly can be answered without exact knowledge of
the absolute minimum requirement, because according to our observations comparison with the vitamin supply parameters of other age groups is valid. Specific
needs for the elderly can arise from:

decreased needs for food and energy
disadvantageous food selection
disturbed digestion
inefficient absorption
diminished retention or storage capacity
increased elimination.

There is an ever-growing body of publications on the vitamin status of the elderly
and on recommended allowances and specific metabolic alterations in old age for
most vitamins. The focus of this chapter is a discussion of the summarized results
of these reports together with the results of a representative nationwide nutrition

---

[a] The minimum requirement of a nutrient is usually considered to be the smallest exogenous supply
needed to prevent symptoms of deficiency, as judged by clinical signs and symptoms and/or by parameters
of biochemical or physiological function (2).

study (the VERA study). The VERA study (5) was carried out on 2006 healthy people aged 18 to 88 years living in private homes in the Federal Republic of Germany in 1987 to 1988 (Tables 1–4). In addition, we have at our disposal the data from 297 very old and multimorbid patients from a geriatric hospital (6) and from two earlier regional nutrition studies, conducted on free-living elderly people (7).

In all these studies vitamin status was determined using comparable biochemical methods, mostly in our own laboratories. A discriminating analysis of the vitamin supply of healthy elderly people and of very old chronically diseased people could thus be made. Even if some details are specific to the nutritional situation in Ger-

TABLE 1. *Vitamin status of the healthy German population (VERA study) and of very old and sick patients in hospital. Medians, 2.5 and 97.5 percentiles (males)*

	Healthy German population (n = 862)			Very old, sick (n = 73)
Age group	18–39 years	40–59 years	60–88 years	75–97 years
Plasma concentrations				
Ascorbic acid	72.7	65.6	61.3	28.4
(μmol/l)	(26.3–108.6)	(20.4–108.5)	(19.3–100.0)	(6.0–71.0)
Folate	13.0	13.0	13.0	
(nmol/l)	(5.0–23.3)	(5.7–26.0)	(6.0–21.2)	
Cobalamin	282.0	276.5	255.0	
(pmol/l)	(126.8–567.6)	(122.0–561.2)	(103.5–426.2)	
Retinol	1.97	2.15	2.03	1.34
(μmol/l)	(1.13–2.85)	(1.31–3.26)	(1.14–3.18)	(0.45–2.90)
β-Carotene	0.44	0.42	0.44	
(μmol/l)	(0.10–1.36)	(0.07–1.29)	(0.11–1.54)	
25(OH)D$_3$	122.0	122.0	147.0	
(nmol/l)	(10.0–800.0)	(10.0–477.4)	(10.0–502.9)	
α-Tocopherol	25.8	31.2	32.1	
(μmol/l)	(16.8–40.6)	(17.6–54.0)	(19.5–55.6)	
Enzyme assays				
α-ETK	1.10	1.11	1.11	1.15
	(1.01–1.20)	(1.02–1.19)	(1.00–1.20)	(1.00–1.42)
α-EGR	1.34	1.31	1.32	1.30
	(1.11–1.64)	(1.13–1.64)	(1.12–1.60)	(1.07–1.82)
α-EAST	1.52	1.51	1.49	1.64
	(1.27–1.85)	(1.23–1.81)	(1.20–1.73)	(1.25–2.23)
Urine concentrations (μmol/24 hr)				
Thiamin	0.93	0.68	0.70	
	(0.14–4.68)	(0.05–6.80)	(0.50–9.93)	
Riboflavin	1.78	1.60	1.42	
	(0.09–7.89)	(0.13–8.38)	(0.11–7.74)	
4-Pyridoxic acid	5.12	5.19	4.84	
	(1.70–25.1)	(1.41–19.5)	(1.54–86.9)	
NMNA	31.2	30.9	28.8	
	(12.6–83.4)	(9.7–79.6)	(9.9–67.2)	

TABLE 2. *Vitamin status of the healthy German population (VERA study) and of very old and sick patients in hospital. Medians, 2.5 and 97.5 percentiles (females)*

	Healthy German population (n = 1144)			Very old, sick (n = 227)
Age group	18–39 years	40–59 years	60–88 years	75–97 years
Plasma concentrations				
Ascorbic acid	80.6	82.3	82.3	38.0
(μmol/l)	(30.1–116.6)	(36.5–114.2)	(29.6–119.0)	(14.0–81.0)
Folate	13.0	13.0	14.0	
(nmol/l)	(2.0–66.0)	(5.7–26.0)	(5.2–31.6)	
Cobalamin	256.5	289.0	271.5	
(pmol/l)	(119.3–526.7)	(110.0–565.0)	(114.5–600.6)	
Retinol	1.75	1.81	1.86	1.44
(μmol/l)	(0.98–2.79)	(1.14–2.86)	(1.15–2.74)	(0.60–3.10)
β-Carotene	0.54	0.66	0.68	
(μmol/l)	(0.14–1.77)	(0.16–1.96)	(0.21–1.99)	
25(OH)D$_3$	132.0	127.0	109.5	
(nmol/l)	(10.0–505.0)	(10.0–448.6)	(10.0–440.6)	
α-Tocopherol	25.7	32.2	34.8	
(μmol/l)	(17.1–39.1)	(20.0–50.4)	(19.0–55.1)	
Enzyme assays				
α-ETK	1.11	1.10	1.10	1.13
	(1.02–1.20)	(1.00–1.19)	(1.01–1.20)	(1.01–1.32)
α-EGR	1.40	1.35	1.30	1.28
	(1.18–1.68)	(1.11–1.66)	(1.08–1.58)	(1.06–1.65)
α-EAST	1.56	1.55	1.57	1.64
	(1.30–1.82)	(1.26–1.85)	(1.20–1.89)	(1.28–2.20)
Urine concentrations (μmol/24 hr)				
Thiamin	0.67	0.69	0.67	
	(0.1–3.25)	(0.11–10.1)	(0.04–9.90)	
Riboflavin	1.30	1.41	1.33	
	(0.10–8.51)	(0.11–8.78)	(0.12–12.2)	
4-Pyridoxic acid	3.54	4.13	4.01	
	(1.09–18.5)	(1.18–14.3)	(1.30–40.0)	
NMNA	26.2	27.5	24.5	
	(8.0–68.6)	(9.7–85.8)	(7.5–102.3)	

many, the conclusions derived from these studies should hold true for other industrialized countries. Since the use of nutrient supplements among the elderly is not nearly as common in many European countries [males: 10%; females: 20% (8)] as in the United States [males: 35%; females: 45% (9)], some of the factors influencing vitamin balance might be more obvious in our particular population groups.

Mean or median values of vitamin parameters in the elderly do not always differ significantly from the younger age groups. Examination of the frequency distribution of the values (Fig. 1) sometimes shows that values obtained from elderly people have a much larger range and often a more skewed distribution than those found in younger

TABLE 3. *Vitamin intake in different age groups of the German population (VERA study),
calculated from a 7-day food record. Medians, 2.5 and 97.5 percentiles (males)*

Age group	Healthy German population (n = 862)		
	18–39 years	40–59 years	60–88 years
Vitamin A	1.02	0.96	1.03
(mg RE)	(0.32–3.48)	(0.34–4.08)	(0.41–3.46)
Carotene	1.49	1.36	1.74
(mg)	(0.34–6.18)	(0.37–5.58)	(0.43–5.59)
Vitamin D	4.07	3.86	3.99
(μg)	(1.1–12.8)	(1.44–12.8)	(1.11–12.5)
Vitamin E	15.9	14.3	14.6
(mg)	(6.8–32.0)	(6.4–28.4)	(7.4–29.4)
Vitamin C	80.5	67.7	78.1
(mg)	(8.0–517.1)	(20.7–211.2)	(19.2–188.5)
Folate	205	195	194.2
(μg)	(99–426)	(109–335)	(105–310)
Vitamin B_{12}	6.0	6.5	5.5
(μg)	(2.43–14.8)	(2.67–16.3)	(2.77–14.2)
Thiamin	1.44	1.34	1.31
(mg)	(0.68–2.63)	(0.71–2.36)	(0.75–1.99)
Riboflavin	1.62	1.66	1.48
(mg)	(0.81–2.90)	(0.87–2.93)	(0.88–2.28)
Vitamin B_6	1.81	1.85	1.76
(mg)	(0.95–2.94)	(1.10–2.98)	(1.05–2.58)

RE, retinol equivalent.

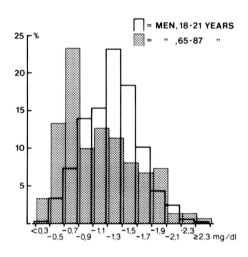

FIG. 1. Plasma concentration of ascorbic acid in a sample of free-living elderly people (n = 317) and young male recruits (n = 1081).

TABLE 4. *Vitamin intake in different age groups of the German population (VERA study), calculated from a 7-day food record. Medians, 2.5 and 97.5 percentiles (females)*

Age group	Healthy German population (n = 1144)		
	18–39 years	40–59 years	60–88 years
Vitamin A	0.85	0.94	0.95
(mg RE)	(0.30–2.73)	(0.32–3.75)	(0.38–2.96)
Carotene	1.51	1.86	1.91
(mg)	(0.33–6.15)	(0.45–6.76)	(0.45–7.07)
Vitamin D	3.10	3.15	3.37
(µg)	(1.0–8.4)	(1.05–10.8)	(0.88–27.3)
Vitamin E	12.7	12.4	13.0
(mg)	(5.2–24.5)	(5.5–24.7)	(5.8–27.9)
Vitamin C	81.9	90.8	95.5
(mg)	(19.4–237.4)	(21.3–236.1)	(27.9–217.7)
Folate	162	167	173
(µg)	(67–314)	(72–290)	(85–308)
Vitamin B_{12}	4.0	4.4	4.3
(µg)	(1.64–10.7)	(1.33–15.9)	(1.95–12.1)
Thiamin	1.07	1.14	1.17
(mg)	(0.53–1.84)	(0.55–1.84)	(0.59–1.81)
Riboflavin	1.30	1.36	1.38
(mg)	(0.58–2.20)	(0.61–2.13)	(0.64–2.36)
Vitamin B_6	1.35	1.49	1.53
(mg)	(0.65–2.20)	(0.68–2.30)	(0.73–2.37)

RE, retinol equivalent.

adults. In some cases differences in the nutrient supplies between different age groups become obvious only when comparing the prevalence of low values (Table 5).

VITAMIN A

The liver is the dominant storage site for vitamin A. In healthy people these stores are normally maintained throughout life (10). There are even data to suggest increased storage with advancing age (11). The assessment of vitamin A supply by measuring plasma retinol concentration is problematic because the plasma level is regulated homeostatically. A decrease in plasma retinol is only obvious when the vitamin A stores of the liver are at least partly depleted. Therefore, a marginal supply cannot be recognized reliably at the plasma level, although early deficiency is characterized by a decrease in concentration of the retinol and retinol-binding protein complex.

The concentration of the retinol-binding protein (RBP) for men and women shows marked differences since it is influenced by hormones. This difference is sustained throughout life. A comparison of the prevalence of low values even shows a lower percentage in the elderly.

No evidence exists of an age-related reduction in vitamin A absorption or a

TABLE 5. *Vitamin status of the healthy German population; prevalence of low values[a]*

Age group		Healthy German population		
		18–39 years (%)	40–59 years (%)	60–88 years (%)
Plasma concentrations				
Ascorbic acid	m	7.6	12.0	15.2
≤36.8 μmol/l	f	3.9	2.3	5.0
Folate	m	4.1	4.1	2.6
≤6.0 nmol/l	f	3.5	3.6	5.3
Cobalamin	m	3.8	3.7	8.7
≤136 pmol/l	f	4.8	2.2	4.3
Retinol				
≤1.34 μmol/l	m	5.6	4.1	3.6
≤1.02 μmol/l	f	3.3	1.4	1.0
β-Carotene	m	10.1	11.9	10.3
≤0.18 μmol/l	f	4.1	3.4	1.5
25(OH)D$_3$	m	6.4	4.9	2.6
≤10 nmol/l	f	5.2	5.0	4.8
α-Tocopherol	m	5.1	2.6	0.5
≤17.7 μmol/l	f	3.9	0.6	1.9
Enzyme assays				
α-ETK	m	4.6	3.0	5.1
≥1.20	f	4.5	4.2	4.4
α-EGR	m	4.3	4.1	3.6
≥1.66	f	5.4	4.5	1.0
α-EAST	m	5.4	3.4	2.1
≥1.85	f	3.7	4.5	6.3

[a] The 2.5 percentiles of a group with sufficient vitamin supplies as indicated by a food frequency were defined as cut-off values.

diminished utilization of the provitamins, providing no chronic intestinal diseases are manifest. Our results correspond to reports from the United States (12), indicating that aged people ingesting the same amounts of vitamin A have the same plasma levels as other adults. Overall, we conclude from this that the recommended vitamin A intake is sufficient.

In contrast to the situation with healthy elderly people, the vitamin A supply of very old geriatric patients shows a marked difference. About 37% of these patients have low plasma retinol concentrations (≤35 mg/dl), whereas in the dangerously ill the prevalence is more than 50%. This finding may not be caused by an insufficient vitamin A intake but by a decrease in RBP concentration.

β-Carotene

The plasma β-carotene concentration is not suitable for characterizing the supply of vitamin A. Based on the inactivation of free radicals, β-carotene, as with other carotenoids, seems to have an additional effect in the organism independent of its function as vitamin A precursor (13). In our study the concentration of β-carotene was analyzed alone. Apart from lycopene, β-carotene is the main component of the carotenoids occurring in plasma. The mean plasma concentration in women is about 40% higher than in men. This can be explained by a sex-specific difference in the elimination of β-carotene (14), in the face of identical carotene intakes. Significant age-related differences were not observed, although the carotene intake seems to increase slightly with age.

VITAMIN D

In our study the plasma concentration of 25-hydroxy-cholecalciferol [25(OH)D$_3$], which is the major form of vitamin D in the plasma, was measured to assess vitamin D status. The vitamin D supply is derived mainly from endogenous vitamin D$_3$ synthesis in the epidermis on exposure to sunlight. If the exposure to sunlight is long enough, no exogenous vitamin D intake is necessary. In sun-poor seasons and in regions with high air pollution, the oral ingestion of vitamin D becomes an important factor for a sufficient vitamin D supply. Therefore, the plasma 25(OH)D$_3$ concentration is primarily an indicator of the average time the person has spent in the open air. Only elderly women show significantly lower plasma 25(OH)D$_3$ concentrations (-30%) with advancing age, especially in winter and spring. In summer and autumn, the vitamin D supply is much better.

There is good evidence that this decrease is caused by a lack of sunlight exposure and not by an age-related impaired hydroxylation in the liver or a less efficient synthesis of vitamin D in the skin (15). Institutionalized or housebound elderly people show lower 25(OH)D$_3$ concentrations than the free-living elderly (16). Therefore, special attention should be paid to a sufficient vitamin D supply for housebound elderly persons throughout the year and for the free-living elderly during the winter and spring months. Under these conditions, vitamin D becomes a real vitamin. Persons regularly consuming sea fish have a significantly better vitamin D status. Since few unfortified foods are rich in vitamin D, a continuous but well controlled supplementation of housebound elderly people might be beneficial.

VITAMIN E

Vitamin E is, in contrast to vitamin D, widely distributed in foods. Moreover, since the organism has a large storage capacity for tocopherol, vitamin E deficiency in man is rare even if the food is relatively unbalanced. Special problems for the assessment of vitamin E status from its plasma concentration arise from the close relation to the blood lipids (17). Since the lipoprotein concentrations and consequently the transport capacity for tocopherols increase with advancing age, mean plasma α-tocopherol concentrations are increased in the elderly. These higher plasma levels do not necessarily indicate higher tissue concentrations. A multiple regression analysis shows that more than 50% of the variation of α-tocopherol in plasma can be explained solely by the variation in the different lipoprotein concentrations. There is no plausible reason for an increased requirement for vitamin E or for increasing the recommendation for the elderly.

VITAMIN K

The minimum requirement of vitamin K is not definitively known. There are neither sufficient data about the vitamin K content of foods nor reliable experimental data about the metabolism of vitamin K in man. Pure diet-induced vitamin K deficiencies in humans are rare (18). Vitamin K deficiency is usually diagnosed by a prolonged prothrombin time or, more recently, by bioanalytical measurement of the vitamin K concentrations in blood. At present, no statement can be made about a specific requirement for vitamin K in the elderly. Since no increased tendency toward hemorrhages in the elderly is known, a sufficient supply of the vitamin can be assumed.

VITAMIN C

The vitamin C supply is usually assessed by measuring the plasma concentration. The plasma ascorbic acid level reacts immediately upon altering the vitamin C intake. The observance of general nutrition guidelines that fresh fruits and vegetables should be eaten daily results in plasma concentrations far above the cut-off value of 12 μmol/l (0.2 mg/dl), which is connected with the appearance of scurvy. Since vitamin C has an important function in protecting the cells against aggressive oxidants, plasma ascorbic acid levels significantly higher than those necessary for the prevention of scurvy seem to be advisable. Sex differences in tubular reabsorption of ascorbic acid in the kidney result in higher mean values for women than for men. Therefore, women have a significant physiological advantage in the supply of this antioxidant vitamin.

In contrast to many other vitamins, comparatively few foods contain significant amounts of vitamin C. In Germany the mean vitamin C intake is about 80 mg/day, and about 10% of Germans seldom eat fresh fruits and vegetables. Extremely low values can be found in persons who eat only bread and butter with marmalade or sausages and drink only tea or coffee. Smokers consume far fewer fruits and vegetables and at the same time require a higher vitamin C intake than non-smokers (19). An age-correlated decline in ascorbic acid levels is observed in men, whereas the mean vitamin C intake shows no corresponding alteration. The women in our study ingested increasing amounts of vitamin C with advancing age. This was without any effect on the plasma levels, because the renal threshold is effective at this high level of intake. Education and income levels and the season are additional factors influencing the vitamin C status of the elderly.

FOLATE

It has been shown in most surveys that average folate intakes are well below the recommended daily allowances. This can partly be explained by incomplete or unreliable folate values in food composition tables and partly by an overgenerous recommendation for the folate intake. Since no deficiency symptoms were evident when consuming somewhat lesser amounts of folate, the recommendations for folate have recently been lowered (4). A linear relationship exists between different folate intakes and plasma folate levels. We could not establish age- or sex-dependent differences in the mean plasma folate concentration. Therefore, healthy elderly people seem to maintain, with advancing age, the ability to hydrolyze folate polyglutamates to folate monoglutamates and to absorb folate at a sufficient rate. Supplementation with folic acid results in a marked increase in plasma folate values. Special attention should be drawn to the influence of drugs, which are commonly taken by aged persons, and alcohol, which might affect folate metabolism and excretion (20). The elderly can be considered to be in the same category as other adults with respect to folate needs.

VITAMIN B_{12}

Animal products are the main dietary sources of vitamin B_{12}. Pernicious anemia is not usually caused by dietary insufficiency, but by disturbed digestion or absorption (21). Vitamin B_{12} deficiency is uncommon even among strict vegetarians and then develops only very slowly. We found that elderly men had significantly lower plasma cobalamin concentrations than younger adults. These findings are consistent with other published data (22). Atrophic gastritis is relatively common among elderly men. This can result in an impaired release of vitamin B_{12} from dietary proteins, due to the lack of gastric acid (23) and a reduced secretion of intrinsic factor. Therefore, elderly people with chronic gastritis should possibly be advised to increase their vitamin B_{12} intake. Storage and enterohepatic circulation of cobalamin seem to be unimpaired.

THIAMIN

The human organism has a relatively low storage capacity for thiamin, so a regular thiamin intake is necessary. In contrast to the RDA (males: 1.2 mg *vs.* 1.5 mg in younger adults), thiamin intake was not reduced in elderly people in Germany. This is consistent with the finding that the intake and the measured status of thiamin do not differ in the aged. The thiamin status was assessed by measuring the activity of the transketolase in erythrocytes (ETK). Thiamin deficiency among healthy adults of all age groups is rare, and different ETK activity coefficients were not obvious. Chronic consumption of alcohol, which affects the absorption and metabolism of thiamin and is accompanied by an insufficient intake of numerous essential nutrients, is the main reason for a thiamin deficiency in the elderly (24). Among very old and sick elderly people the prevalence of low values increases significantly. There is no evidence to justify a specific additional need for thiamin in the elderly.

RIBOFLAVIN

Milk and milk products, which are the most important source of riboflavin, are less frequently consumed by the elderly. Nevertheless, non-milk drinkers can achieve the recommendation for riboflavin without any difficulty through other riboflavin sources. The assessment of riboflavin status by glutathione-reductase activity in erythrocytes (EGR) reveals no age-related influence, although the riboflavin intake declines significantly with advancing age. This indicates that despite the decreased riboflavin intake—as reflected by a lower riboflavin excretion in urine—the riboflavin supply is sufficient on the cellular level. Since no definitive evidence for an age-related alteration of riboflavin metabolism exists, it can be concluded that the riboflavin requirement is not affected by aging.

VITAMIN B$_6$

Vitamin B$_6$ is widely distributed in foods. In our population study the vitamin B$_6$ supply was assessed by measuring the aspartate-aminotransferase activity in erythrocytes (EAST) and the excretion of 4-pyridoxic acid in urine. The median values of EAST activity coefficients indicate no age-related differences. The comparison of the prevalence of low α-EAST values shows that the percentage of such values, indicating an insufficient vitamin B$_6$ supply, increases with advancing age in women. A possible interaction should be considered between vitamin B$_6$ and drugs containing estrogens, which are frequently prescribed to elderly women in the prophylaxis of osteoporosis. Since there are also published reports describing an age-related decrease in pyridoxol-5-phosphate (PLP) concentration, an age-dependent alteration in vitamin B$_6$ metabolism cannot be excluded. Very old and sick people have a much more unfavorable vitamin B$_6$ supply. At present, however, data from animal experiments and human trials are not sufficient to alter the recommendations for vitamin B$_6$ in elderly people.

NIACIN

The assessment of niacin supply is extraordinarily difficult, since a reliable calculation of ingested niacin on the basis of the incomplete data that exist at present is impossible. For the assessment of niacin status, only the urinary excretion of niacin metabolites is available. A more reliable index is still to be found. Compared with middle-aged persons, we found a decline of the *N*-methyl-nicotinamide (NMNA) excretion (-10%) in the elderly. This raises no cause for concern, as the excretion of NMNA indicates that the niacin supply in the whole population is more than adequate. Since less energy and protein are required in old age, dietary reasons for the decline in NMNA excretion can be assumed. There is no basis for the assumption that the conversion from tryptophan to niacin is impaired in the elderly. A further estimation of a specific need for niacin in the aged cannot be made at the present time.

BIOTIN

As with other B vitamins, biotin is widely distributed in foods. The biotin intake shows a wide variation and biotin from intestinal bacterial synthesis seems to be available. Therefore, biotin deficiency in man is rare. In most national recommendations no data for biotin have been established. Until recently a reliable biochemical method was not available. Since the few data existing are limited and moreover contradictory, further consideration would be speculative at the moment.

PANTOTHENIC ACID

No specific pantothenic acid deficiency symptoms have reliably been described up to now. Pantothenic acid is widely distributed among foods. Data about the pantothenic acid supply of the population are fragmentary. The obvious absence of pantothenic acid deficiency in man might be due to the wide distribution of this vitamin in foods. No agreement has been reached on the age-dependency of pantothenic acid concentrations in plasma (25). A conclusion about specific needs for the elderly cannot be drawn.

CONCLUSION

At the same intake levels, the vitamin supply parameters of elderly persons do not vary from those of young persons. An exception may possibly occur in the case of vitamin C and vitamin B_{12} for men. This should be subject to further investigations. The currently available data do not allow the definitive conclusion that there is an age-specific vitamin requirement. The insufficient vitamin status of very old multimorbid patients is more a result of accompanying sicknesses than of old age per se. This insufficient vitamin status is, however, cause for concern and requires more therapeutic attention than is currently given.

In earlier studies, we could show that marginal vitamin deficiencies in elderly persons were accompanied by objective psychological disorders (26). These findings have now been confirmed in studies on younger adults, provided the marginal deficiency was not merely short-term (27).

It should not be forgotten that even though the average vitamin supply of the elderly in our studies was surprisingly good, persons with poor education, low in-

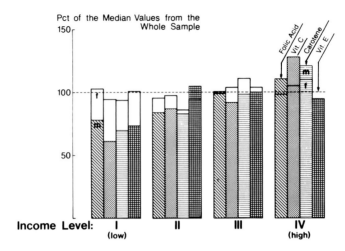

FIG. 2. Vitamin status and income level. Pct, percent.

come (Fig. 2), and of high consumption of alcohol, cigarettes, and drugs show significantly increased risk of low values.

ACKNOWLEDGMENTS

The VERA study was supported by the Ministry for Research and Technology of the Federal Republic of Germany, grant 704752 and 704754. The authors are responsible for the content of this publication. We thank Falayi Adu for his assistance in preparing the manuscript.

REFERENCES

1. Beaton GH. Toward harmonization of dietary, biochemical, and clinical assessments: the meanings of nutritional status and requirements. *Nutr Rev* 1986;44:349–58.
2. FAO/WHO. Requirements of ascorbic acid, vitamin D, vitamin B_{12}, folate, and iron. Report of a Joint FAO/WHO Expert Group. *WHO Tech Rep Ser* 1970;452:22–5.
3. Deutsche Gesellschaft für Ernährung. *Empfehlungen für die Nährstoffzufuhr*. Frankfurt: Umschau Verlag, 1991.
4. National Research Council. *Recommended dietary allowances*. 10th ed. Washington, DC: National Academy Press, 1989.
5. Heseker H, Kohlmeier M, Schneider R, Speitling A, Kübler W. Vitaminversorgung Erwachsener in der Bundesrepublik Deutschland. *Ernährungs-Umschau* 1991;38:227–33.
6. Volkert D, Frauenrath C, Kruse W, Oster P, Schlierf G. Ernährungszustand geriatrischer Patienten. In: Schmitz-Scherzer R, Kurse A, Olbrich E, eds. *Altern—Ein lebenslanger Prozeß der sozialen Interaktion*. Darmstadt: Steinkopff–Verlag, 1990:117–26.
7. Heseker H, Kübler W. Die Bedarfsdeckung älterer Menschen mit Vitaminen. *Ernährungs-Umschau* 1983;30:366–9.
8. Gregory J, Foster K, Tyler H, Wiseman M. *The dietary and nutritional survey of British adults*. London: HMSO, 1990.

9. Hale WE, Stewart RB, Cerda JJ, Marks RG, May FE. Use of nutritional supplements in an ambulatory elderly population. *J Am Geriatr Soc* 1982;30:401–3.
10. Hoppner K, Phillips WEJ, Murray TK, Campbell JS. Survey of liver vitamin A stores of Canadians. *Can Med Assoc J* 1968;99:983–6.
11. Underwood BA, Siegel H, Weisell RC, Dolinsky M. Liver stores of vitamin A in a normal population dying suddenly or rapidly from unnatural causes in New York City. *Am J Clin Nutr* 1970;23: 1037–42.
12. Garry PJ, Hunt WC, Bandrofchak JL, VanderJagt DJ, Goodwin JS. Vitamin A intake and plasma retinol levels in healthy elderly men and women. *Am J Clin Nutr* 1987;46:989–94.
13. DiMascio P, Murphy ME, Sies H. Antioxidant defense systems: the role of carotenoids, tocopherols, and thiols. *Am J Clin Nutr* 1991;53:194–200S.
14. Kübler W. Pharmocokinetic implications of single and repeated dosage. In: Walter P, Stähelin H, Brubacher G, eds. *Elevated dosages of vitamins*. Toronto: Hans Huber Publishers, 1989:25–34.
15. Munro HN, Suter PM, Russell RM. Nutritional requirements of the elderly. *Annu Rev Nutr* 1987;7: 23–49.
16. Vir SC, Love AHG. Vitamin D status of elderly at home and non-institutionalized aged in hospital. *Int J Vitamin Res* 1978;48:123–30.
17. Burton GW, Traber MG. Vitamin E: antioxidant activity, biokinetics, and bioavailability. *Annu Rev Nutr* 1990;10:357–82.
18. Suttie JW. Vitamin K. In: Machlin LJ, ed. *Handbook of vitamins*. 2nd ed. New York: Marcel Dekker, 1991:145–94.
19. Kallner AB, Hartmann D, Hornig DH. On the requirements of ascorbic acid in man: steady-state turnover and body-pool in smokers. *Am J Clin Nutr* 1981;34:1347–55.
20. Rosenberg IH, Bowman BB, Cooper BA, Halsted CH, Lindenbaum J. Folate nutrition in the elderly. *Am J Clin Nutr* 1982;36:1060–66.
21. Herbert V. Vitamin B_{12}. In: *Present knowledge in nutrition*. 5th ed. Washington, DC: The Nutrition Foundation, 1984:347–64.
22. Suter PM, Russell RL. Vitamin requirements of the elderly. *Am J Clin Nutr* 1987;45:501–12.
23. King CE, Leibach J, Toskes PP. Clinically significant vitamin B_{12} deficiency secondary to malabsorption of protein-bound vitamin B_{12}. *Dig Dis Sci* 1979;24:397–402.
24. Iber FI, Blass JP, Brin M, Leevy CM. Thiamin in the elderly—relation to alcoholism and to neurological degenerative disease. *Am J Clin Nutr* 1982;36:1067–82.
25. Srinivasan V, Christensen N, Wyse BW, Hansen RG. Pantothenic acid nutritional status in the elderly—institutionalized and noninstitutionalized. *Am J Clin Nutr* 1981;34:1736–42.
26. Chome J, Paul T, Pudel V, *et al.* Effects of suboptimal vitamin status on behavior. *Bibl Nutr Dieta* 1986;38:94–103.
27. Heseker H, Kübler W, Westenhöfer J, Pudel V. Psychische Veränderungen als Frühzeichen einer suboptimalen Vitaminversorgung. *Ernährungs-Umschau* 1990;37:87–94.

DISCUSSION

Dr. Chandra: I have a general question about the way in which we define deficiency of a vitamin. If you use a cut-off point, say the 2.5 percentile, based on individuals whose intakes are considered normal, how can you be sure it is appropriate? I think "normal" in this context is describing the average intake rather than the normal or healthy intake. Unless we can look at some nutrition-specific *function*, and unfortunately we do not have many of these, I do not think we can be sure we are measuring deficiency. I suspect the incidence of deficiency is higher than we think.

Dr. Heseker: This is a big unsolved problem. It is impossible to use cut-off values from the literature because the methodological variations are so great. There is at present in Europe a program to obtain standard cut-off values from different laboratories. Different institutes are working on this and all receive the same samples to analyze so that the values can be standardized. In our study we defined reference values from a reference population. This consisted of people between the ages of 18 and 65 years, none of them overweight, and none smoking more than 10 cigarettes a day or drinking more than half a liter of beer a day. The sample comprised about 200 people and we used the 2.5 percentile as the reference value. I can say with confidence that the values under this cut-off represent a higher risk of deficiency. I think it is better to have such a cut-off than to have no cut-off at all. However, a lot of work has to be done in this field and functional tests have to be developed.

Dr. Guesry: We should not have the same definitions of vitamin deficiency as we had 200 years ago. The role of vitamin C is no longer to prevent scurvy, and while the role of vitamin A is still to prevent xerophthalmia in developing countries, in Western societies its importance in the elderly is probably more related to its antioxidant role. I think we need new definitions of the requirements for vitamins. As an example, don't you think that if we are recommending an increased intake of polyunsaturated fatty acids, and especially linoleic acid, we should increase the recommended intake of vitamin E, which stabilizes membranes in the presence of excess linoleic acid? Similarly for vitamin C: we are increasingly recommending the use of soya protein, which decreases iron absorption; we know that vitamin C counterbalances this decrease in iron absorption, so we should reconsider our recommendations for vitamin C intake under these circumstances. I think we need to reconsider vitamin requirements with a new vision.

Dr. Heseker: I think our cut-off values are already a move in this direction. For example, our value for α-tocopherol is about 700 μg/dl, and the normally quoted value is much lower. Our cut-off value for vitamin C is 0.7 mg/dl, which is a very high value. The question of the recommended vitamin C intake is an interesting one. Should we recommend an intake at which the tissues are saturated with vitamin C, for example? If so, we need an intake of about 100 mg per day, at which level the plasma concentrations will be about 1 mg/dl; or do we look at the level necessary to prevent scurvy?

Dr. Bowman: Various surveys continue to show that vitamin B_6 is a problem nutrient for the elderly. A paper published by a Dutch group recently (1) suggests that B_6 requirements may be significantly higher for the elderly, and a very recent paper reports significantly higher vitamin B_6 requirements in healthy elderly Americans (2). Could you comment?

Dr. Heseker: In our relatively healthy population of elderly people, the vitamin B_6 status was good. I believe that B_6 supply is not a problem if a good variety of foods is consumed. You have to have a very unbalanced diet to get insufficient B_6. When we find low values, they are usually in very old and ill people and in those on restricted diets.

Dr. van Staveren: In The Netherlands vitamin B_6 is a real problem. I think it would be nice to compare data because we find systematically low values and I don't think the diets are so abnormal.

Dr. Munro: Studies were done some 10 years ago comparing nursing home patients in New Jersey and in Northern Ireland with the free-living population. Different patterns were found for the various vitamins that were measured. In some cases you do better in a nursing home in New Jersey, in others you do better in Belfast. The different patterns presumably reflect differences in the intakes of vitamins related to the local food supplies. They do not necessarily indicate that low levels are clinically important. I believe that until you can obtain clinical data as well as blood levels and possibly dietary intakes, you cannot really arrive at conclusions that can justifiably be used to reverse government policies or the recommendations of other agencies.

Dr. Heseker: I know these studies. I think some of the discrepancies might have been due to the problem of cut-off values. We did our first study of elderly people in 1980–1981 and we found a higher proportion with low values than we find now, in keeping with there being a better vitamin supply now than there was 10 years ago. I think the mean vitamin supply for the population has never been as good as it is today. The main problem in the future will be to increase the vitamin supply of those people who do not take care of their health and nutrition. People with a well balanced diet eat also a lot of fruits and vegetables, drink fruit juices, and also use vitamin supplements. This means the ones who would really need additional vitamins don't use the different possibilities.

REFERENCES

1. Löwick MRH, Schrijver J, Odink J, van den Berg H, Wedel M, Hermus RJJ. Nutrition and aging: nutritional status of "apparently healthy" elderly (Dutch Nutrition Surveillance System). *J Am Coll Nutr* 1990;9(1):18–27.
2. Ribaya-Mercado JD, Russell RM, Sahyoun N, Morrow FD, Gershoff SN. Vitamin B_6 requirements of the elderly men and women. *J Nutr* 1991;12:1062–74.

Nutrition of the Elderly, edited by H. Munro and
G. Schlierf, Nestlé Nutrition Workshop Series, Vol. 29,
Nestec Ltd., Vevey/Raven Press, Ltd., New York 1992.

Trace Elements in Aging

Walter Mertz

Beltsville Human Nutrition Research Center, Agricultural Research Service, USDA,
Beltsville, Maryland 20705, USA

Knowledge of mineral element status and requirements in older people is incomplete and, for most elements, derived by extrapolation from younger age groups. Yet some valid conclusions can be drawn on the basis of known age-related changes in body composition, in energy needs, and in food intake to meet these requirements. In the following discussion I shall first deal with iron, the requirement for which changes abruptly in women with menopause, and then I shall deal with other elements, according to their changes in concentration in the human body through life.

IRON

The requirement for iron is sharply reduced in postmenopausal women, and their iron nutrition is correspondingly improved (1). Iron has special nutritional interest because of the high incidence of iron deficiency worldwide in infants, children, adolescents, and women. Because the biological availability of dietary iron depends heavily on the composition of the diet eaten, dietary recommendations vary according to the nature of the national diet. An Expert Consultation of the Food and Agricultural Organization/World Health Organization (2) set a median requirement to prevent anemia in women of childbearing age at 17, 8, and 5.6 mg per day for diets of low, intermediate, and high iron bioavailability. These high recommendations, difficult to implement in all but high bioavailability diets, are sharply reduced in postmenopausal women, to 10, 6.5, and 3.4 mg, respectively. These amounts are easily obtained from almost all diets; consequently, iron status of postmenopausal women improves markedly. Because adult men generally have no problem in meeting their iron requirements, it can be stated that as a general rule iron status improves as people get older. Anemia in older individuals is rarely caused by iron deficiency; when it occurs, chronic blood loss or deficiency of folacin or vitamin B_{12} should be looked for. Whether iron plays a substantial role in the aging process is not known. As is true for most essential elements, iron is required for normal functioning of the immune system; on the other hand, high iron stores in relation to levels of other essential elements have been implicated as risk factors in malnourished children (3), as well as in adults with hemochromatosis. Therefore, concern about the iron status of older people should rather be with the avoidance of overexposure than with the prevention of deficiency.

OTHER TRACE ELEMENTS

For other trace elements, including fluorine, manganese, copper, zinc, selenium, molybdenum, and iodine, there is either direct knowledge that tissue concentrations remain steady during life or a lack of data suggesting consistent changes. Of these elements, all except manganese and molybdenum may present problems of nutritional deficiencies in some parts of the world, and these have led to corrective public health measures (4). It must be noted, however, that by far the greatest risk of deficiency for these elements is found during the early periods of life, including intrauterine development, rather than in old age. Dietary copper deficiency has been described only in children, growth retardation and dwarfism due to zinc deficiency between infancy and adolescence, Keshan disease in children and young pregnant women, and the deleterious effects of lack of fluorine on dental health only during the years during which the permanent teeth are formed. There is no information indicating similar deficiencies in older people.

PHYSIOLOGICAL REQUIREMENT FOR TRACE ELEMENTS DURING AGING

The trace element nutritional status of older people may be jeopardized by the decline in total food intake and by the decreasing efficiency of intestinal absorption, especially in areas where the concentration of essential elements in the diet and in the environment is marginal. On the other hand, the reduction in food intake is often accompanied by a reduction in lean body mass (5), resulting in physiological reduction in the pool size for trace elements. To maintain a reduced pool size requires a smaller intake than would be necessary to maintain a larger pool. The fact that there is no evidence for a substantial decline in tissue concentrations of the elements with age suggests that age *per se* does not jeopardize the trace element status. Neither does it protect against inadequate intakes of elements that are marginal at other ages. Therefore, the adequacy of selenium or iodine intake in the various low-selenium or low-iodine areas of the world, and the adequacy of copper and zinc intake from diets of predominant cereal origin, should remain a matter of concern, regardless of age.

IMMUNE FUNCTION

The physiological functions of elements such as copper, zinc, and iron deserve special study because of their relevance to aspects of the aging process. All three elements are essential for proper functioning of many components of immune defense

(6). Judging from animal experiments, the requirement to maintain optimal immune function appears to be greater than that needed for prevention of the other well established signs of deficiency (7). The function of the immune system is known to decline with age, but convincing data for a protective effect of supplementation with any one trace element in humans are still sparse.

Manganese, copper, zinc, and selenium, in addition, play essential roles in the antioxidant defense system through their function in superoxide dismutases and glutathione peroxidase (4). Since free-radical damage to cellular constituents has been hypothesized as one process responsible for aging, it could be postulated that a deficiency of any of these elements might hasten the aging process. There are, however, no solid data that would indicate a decline in the enzyme functions discussed above.

TOXICITY OF TRACE ELEMENTS DURING AGING

Although the organism has effective mechanisms protecting against accumulation of most essential elements, the protection is relatively weak against accumulation of the anionic forms in which fluorine, iodine, selenium, and molybdenum often occur. Toxic accumulation of all of those is known, reflecting excessive concentrations in the geochemical environment. Here again, the medical consequences are much more important for the young than for the older age groups.

Under conditions that might exist in many industrialized societies, three elements, fluorine, lead, and cadmium, are known to accumulate in human tissues with increasing age. Except for greatly excessive exposure, fluorine and lead are deposited in the bones and pose no particular health problem to the aging organism. Cadmium, on the other hand, accumulates predominantly in the kidney and has been connected with declining renal function (4).

The biological actions of arsenic and mercury depend on their chemical forms and on their interactions with the essential trace element selenium (4). Historically, it is well known that the slow accumulation of low doses of arsenic not only creates a tolerance against higher doses but is also claimed to confer increased physical performance in both man and animals. Arsenic toxicity is known only from criminal, accidental, or very occasionally environmental overexposure. An example of the first was the wide use of arsenic as a poison during the Middle Ages; of the second, the accidental use for human consumption of the arsenic-treated seeds in Iraq some years ago; and of the third, the consumption of drinking water contaminated with arsenic in Argentina, Chile, Mexico, and Taiwan (4). It is unlikely that under most normal circumstances arsenic presents a health problem specifically to the aging organism.

The toxicity of mercury depends strongly on its valency state and on its chemical form (4). A methylated form, methyl mercury, has a high affinity for the central nervous system and is very toxic. On the other hand, poorly defined forms, such as compounds of selenium and mercury, which occur in nature, are believed to be practically inert. Because many natural sources of dietary mercury contain the mercury–selenium combination, mercury is not believed to be an exceptional hazard to the aging organism. For this element, as with many others, it is important to judge toxicity not by simple analytical values but by data based on speciation.

CHROMIUM AND SILICON: POSSIBLE AGE-RELATED DEFICIENCY

Two essential elements, chromium and silicon, appear to decline with age in human tissues, although much more is known about chromium than about silicon. A thorough analytical study by Schroeder *et al.* demonstrated a gradual decline in chromium in human autopsy material from industrialized societies, although not in the lungs in which that element accumulates (8). Livers from diabetics contain less chromium than those from healthy subjects and aortas from patients who died from heart disease less than those of normal individuals. Chromium has been defined as a cofactor for the interaction of insulin with its tissue receptors; chromium deficiency in humans and experimental animals results in a relative insulin resistance that manifests itself by impaired glucose tolerance in the presence of normal or even increased insulin concentrations (4,9). It has been postulated that chromium deficiency contributes to the gradual decline in glucose tolerance with age in the great majority of people living in the United States. A safe and adequate range of dietary chromium intake has been recommended at between 50 and 200 μg per day (10); the minimum requirement for adults can be estimated at between 25 and 30 μg. This amount is not always furnished by typical Western-style diets, especially those high in refined products. Experimental diets furnishing between 15 and 20 μg per day to human volunteers with slightly impaired glucose tolerance have produced a progressive further impairment of glucose tolerance in the presence of gradually increasing serum insulin concentrations, changes that were reversed by daily supplementation with 200 μg of chromium (11). Because impaired glucose tolerance and raised circulating insulin levels are independent risk factors for cardiovascular disease (12), it is possible that chromium deficiency may be contributing a significant risk to that group of disorders. Although chromium deficiency has been described in malnourished children and in patients on low chromium total parenteral nutrition (4), the predominant public health importance of that element lies with the large number of older people with impaired glucose tolerance. Intervention studies on a large scale in older people promise to produce tangible benefits.

Much less is known about the biochemical role, metabolism, and requirement of silicon (4). Its essentiality for bone health has been established independently in rats and chickens. Both species develop gross bone deformities when raised on low silicon diets (1–7 μg/g), associated with abnormalities in the formation of cartilage and connective tissue in general. The requirement for the prevention of these signs may lie between 50 and 250 μg of soluble Si/g diet (4).

Silicon appears to decline with age in the aortas of human subjects, as well as in aortas affected by atherosclerosis (13). A requirement for man has not been established; thus, it is not known whether the habitual intake from Western-type diets of 20 to 50 mg/day is adequate, or whether higher intakes might maintain tissue concentrations. In view of the role of silicon in bone formation and in connective tissue metabolism in general, its accumulation in the brain of patients with Alzheimer's disease, and its potential carcinogenicity in the form of special insoluble compounds such as asbestos, human studies of the metabolism, mode of action, and requirement of silicon are of high priority.

REFERENCES

1. Morris ER. Iron. In: Mertz W, ed. *Trace elements in human and animal nutrition.* 5th ed, Vol II. San Diego: Academic Press, 1987:79–142.
2. Joint FAO/WHO Expert Consultation. *Requirements of vitamin A, iron, folate and vitamin B$_{12}$.* Rome: FAO, 1988.
3. Golden MHN, Golden BE, Bennett FI. Relationship of trace element deficiencies to malnutrition. In: Chandra RK, ed. *Trace elements in nutrition of children.* New York: Raven Press, 1985: 185–207.
4. Mertz W, ed. *Trace elements in human and animal nutrition.* 5th ed, vols I and II. San Diego: Academic Press, 1986, 1987.
5. Munro HN. Protein nutriture and requirements of the elderly. In: Munro HN, Danford DE, eds. *Nutrition, aging and the elderly.* New York: Plenum Press, 1989:153–81.
6. Chandra RK. Trace elements and immune responses. In: Chandra RK, ed. *Trace elements in nutrition of children II.* New York: Raven Press, 1991:201–14.
7. Babu U, Failla ML. Copper status and function of neutrophils are reversibly depressed in marginally and severely copper-deficient rats. *J Nutr* 1990;120:1700–9.
8. Schroeder HA, Balassa JJ, Tipton IH. Abnormal trace metals in man—chromium. *J Chron Dis* 1962;15:941–64.
9. International Programme on Chemical Safety. *Chromium. Environmental Health Criteria 61.* Geneva: World Health Organization, 1988.
10. Food and Nutrition Board. *Recommended dietary allowances.* 10th ed. Washington, DC: National Academy Press, 1989.
11. Anderson RA, Polansky MM, Bryden NA, et al. Supplemental chromiun effects on glucose, insulin, glucagon, and urinary chromium losses in subjects consuming controlled low-chromium diets. *Am J Clin Nutr* 1991;54:909–16.
12. Stout RW. The relationship of abnormal circulating insulin levels to atherosclerosis. *Atherosclerosis* 1977;27:1–13.
13. Loeper J, Loeper J, Fragny M. The physiological role of the silicon and its antiatheromatous action. In: Bends G, Lindquist I, eds. *Biochemistry of silicon and related problems.* New York: Plenum, 1978:281–306.

DISCUSSION

Dr. Kritchevsky: Could you cite the data that now make arsenic essential?

Dr. Mertz: The data come from F.H. Nielsen in Grand Forks, North Dakota, who is working with chickens and rats and from Manfred Anke in Jena, Germany, who uses minipigs and goats. References in two good review articles by these authors are given below (1,2).

REFERENCES

1. Anke M, Krause U, Groppel B. The effect of arsenic deficiency on growth, reproduction, life expectancy and disease symptoms in animals. In: Hemphill DD, ed. *Trace substances in environmental health—21.* Columbia, MO: University of Missouri, 1987:533–50.
2. Nielsen FH. Ultratrace elements in nutrition. *Annu Rev Nutr* 1984;4:21–41.

Nutrition of the Elderly, edited by H. Munro, and
G. Schlierf, Nestlé Nutrition Workshop Series, Vol. 29,
Nestec Ltd., Vevey/Raven Press, Ltd., New York © 1992.

Hip Fracture, Femoral Bone Mineral Density, and Protein Supply in Elderly Patients

Jean-Philippe Bonjour, Charles-Henri Rapin, René Rizzoli,
Lubos Tkatch, Marino Delmi, Thierry Chevalley,
Verena Nydegger, Daniel Slosman, and Harold Vasey

*Division of Clinical Pathophysiology, Department of Medicine; University Institute of
Geriatrics; Division of Nuclear Medicine, Department of Radiology; Orthopaedic
Clinic, Department of Surgery, University Hospital,
CH-1211 Geneva, Switzerland*

Osteoporosis is widely recognized as a major problem in public health. The most dramatic expression of this disease is represented by fractures of the proximal femur. In this chapter we shall consider the problem of malnutrition that can be observed in elderly patients with hip fracture and present two prospective studies indicating that daily oral dietary supplementation providing an adequate intake of protein can substantially improve the clinical course. However, before discussing our investigations on nutritional aspects, it seems appropriate to present briefly the magnitude of the hip fracture problem in our area and its relation to femoral mineral density, since malnutrition is considered as a risk factor in the maintenance of bone mass during adult life.

EPIDEMIOLOGICAL ASPECTS

Several studies (1–6) indicate that the number of hospital admissions of elderly patients with proximal femur fractures has increased considerably during the last 20 years. The same trend was observed in the University Hospital of Geneva (Switzerland). This prompted us to investigate (7) the incidence of all hip fractures as well as of those most likely to be due to osteoporosis, and the coinciding medical and social conditions, in the region of Geneva, which has the oldest population in Switzerland. The Geneva region seemed to be well suited to this kind of epidemiological study, since more than 90% of the patients with hip fractures are referred to one center, allowing a homogeneous evaluation. During 1987, 361 patients with hip fracture were recorded in the University of Geneva hospital, which is the main referral center for a population of about 376,000 inhabitants. This represented 94% of all hip fractures occurring in the region. Moderate trauma was reported in 329 cases (91.1%). The overall annual incidence was 96.1 per 100,000 population (146.9 for women and 39.8 for men). When only hip fractures following moderate trauma were considered, the incidence was 87.6 per 100,000 population (138.8 for women and 30.8 for men). Rare under the age of 65, hip fracture incidence increased exponentially later on. The mean age of patients with hip fracture was 82.0 in women and 75.7 years in men. The mean length of stay in the orthopedic ward was 30.5 days. During the stay in the orthopedic ward the mortality rate was 8.2% and about 55% of the patients displayed one or more severe complications such as bedsore, pneumonia, or pyelonephritis. The costs amounted to 8.8 million Swiss francs for hip fracture associated with moderate trauma. Forty-seven percent of subjects were transferred to another hospital for recovery or rehabilitation. Therefore, the overall cost of hospital admission exceeded 10 million Swiss francs. This survey emphasizes the high incidence and economic importance of hip fractures in a region of Switzerland where the population is particularly old. The problem will probably worsen with the progressive aging of the population. Therefore, it appears appropriate to study factors that could affect both the incidence of hip fractures and their dramatic consequences on the health of the elderly and on the economic burden of medical services in our region.

RELATION BETWEEN FEMORAL BONE MINERAL DENSITY AND HIP FRACTURE

Hip fracture incidence depends on several factors such as the propensity to fall and the insufficiency of protective mechanisms such as reaction time and muscle strength, which may decrease the force required to fracture a piece of the skeleton (8.9). It also depends on specific bone properties such as bone mass and bone architecture. As the breaking strength of bone is directly proportional to bone density (10,11), age-related bone loss should be a major determinant of the risk of fracture. Thus, the incidence of hip fracture has been found to be inversely correlated with femoral neck bone mineral content (12). However, direct determination of bone mineral density of the femoral neck has failed to show a significant difference between patients with hip fracture and age-matched normal individuals in some studies (13,14), but not in others (15,16). An interval between fracture and bone mineral density measurement of up to 5 years might have precluded the detection of a difference. Indeed, either overloading of the contralateral limb or undermobilization during the period following the fracture might have caused an increase or a decrease in femoral neck mineral density. In order to clarify this important issue, we measured bone mineral density in the femoral neck on the opposite side to the fracture, as well as in the femoral shaft and in the lumbar spine (L2–L4), by dual photon absorptiometry (17) in 68 patients (57 women and 11 men, mean age 78.8 ± 1.0 years, mean ± SEM) 12.4 ± 0.8 days after hip fracture following a moderate trauma (18). These values were compared to mineral density at the same bone sites in 93 non-fractured elderly control subjects (82 women and 11 men) measured during the same period. As compared with the controls, femoral neck bone mineral density was significantly lower in women with fractures (0.592 ± 0.013 *vs.* 0.728 ± 0.014 g/cm^2, $p < 0.001$) and also in men with fractures (0.697 ± 0.029 *vs.* 0.840 ± 0.052, $p < 0.05$). Expressed as standard deviations above or below the mean bone mineral density of age- and sex-matched normal subjects (Z score), the difference in femoral neck bone mineral density between women with fractures and controls was highly significant ($-0.6 ± 0.1$ *vs.* $+0.1 ± 0.1$, $p < 0.001$). As compared with mean value in young normal subjects, bone mineral density was decreased by 36.9 ± 1.4 and 22.4 ± 1.5% ($p < 0.001$) in women with fractures and controls, respectively. Femoral neck bone mineral density was lower than 0.705 g/cm^2 in 90% of the women with fractures. The prevalence of fracture increased with decreasing bone density, reaching 100% with values below 0.500 g/cm^2. Femoral shaft and L2–L4 bone mineral densities were significantly lower in women with hip fractures than in controls (1.388 ± 0.036 *vs.* 1.580 ± 0.030, $p < 0.001$, for femoral shaft; and 0.886 ± 0.027 *vs.* 0.985 ± 0.023, $p < 0.01$, for L2–L4), but these differences were not significant when expressed as a Z score. In men with a recent hip fracture, femoral shaft bone density was significantly lower than in controls (1.729 ± 0.096 *vs.* 2.069 ± 0.062, $p < 0.01$), but the difference at the lumbar spine level did not reach statistical significance. These results indicate that both women and men with a recent hip fracture had decreased bone mineral density of the femoral neck, femoral shaft, and lumbar spine. However, the difference appeared to be of greater magnitude in the femoral neck, suggesting a preferential bone loss at this site (18).

RELATION BETWEEN NUTRITION AND HIP FRACTURE

Malnutrition may well represent an important determinant of both incidence and complications of hip fractures in the elderly. The aging population is known to present a high prevalence of malnutrition and patients with fracture of proximal femur appear particularly undernourished, as pointed out by several authors (19–22). Therefore, malnutrition can be considered as a risk factor for hip fracture. Several reasons have been proposed to support this contention. First, malnutrition can be expected to accelerate the process of age-dependent bone loss, since diets deficient in calcium and/or protein are often associated with osteoporosis. Second, malnutrition can be expected to increase the propensity to fall by impairing the coordination of movements (23). Finally, malnutrition could affect the above-mentioned protective mechanisms, such as reaction time and muscle strength, which may decrease the power of impact required to fracture an osteoporotic hip (8,9). After the occurrence of the fracture, nutritional deficiencies may lead to an increase in complications and a greater mortality rate. It has been reported that either supplementary nasogastric tube feeding (24) or parenteral nutrition (25) may be associated with an improvement in clinical outcome following femoral neck fracture in elderly subjects.

BENEFITS OF ORAL DIETARY SUPPLEMENT ON CLINICAL OUTCOME IN PATIENTS WITH HIP FRACTURE

In an initial prospective randomized study (26) we assessed the clinical benefits of a simple oral dietary supplement taken by elderly patients after fracture of the proximal femur. The effects on clinical evolution of a simple dietary intervention provided as an oral protein-energy supplement were studied in elderly patients with femoral neck fractures due to moderate trauma.

Patients and Dietary Supplementation

Fifty-nine patients, mean age 82 years, were randomized in two groups when entering the orthopedic clinic. Twenty-seven patients received a daily oral nutritional supplement, in addition to the standard hospital diet. Thirty-two patients were used as controls. The oral nutritional supplement provided 254 kcal, 20.4 g protein, 29.5 g carbohydrate, 5.8 g lipid, 525 mg calcium, 750 IU vitamin A, 25 IU vitamin D_3, vitamins E, B_1, B_2, B_6, B_{12}, C, nicotinamide, folate, calcium-pantothenate, biotin, and minerals in 250 ml. It was started on admission to the orthopedic clinic and continued throughout the stay in the second (recovery) hospital. The supplement was given at 8 PM, so that it did not interfere with the scheduled meals, for a mean period of 32 days. It was well accepted, completely ingested, and no side effects were observed.

Nutritional Deficiencies on Admission

Anthropometric and biochemical evaluation confirmed the presence of nutritional deficiencies in a majority of patients on admission (19–22). Mean plasma concentration of 25-hydroxyvitamin D of the total study population was 18.9 nmol/l, below the lower limit of normal range (23 nmol/l), with as many as 80% of the subjects displaying poor vitamin D status. The mean concentrations of several nutritional indicators such as retinol-binding protein, vitamin A, and carotene were also below the normal range. This expression of undernutrition appeared to be more severe than that observed among the general aging population (19–22). It cannot be explained by one single cause, since medical, psychological, social, ethnic, and environmental factors probably play an intricate role.

Inadequate Food Intake During Hospital Stay

A precise dietary survey based on 50 daily determinations of the food intake, as assessed by the weighing method, confirmed that nutritional requirements were not covered while the patients were staying in the hospital, despite adequate quantities offered. The voluntary oral intake of energy was only 1,100 ± 300 kcal/day (mean

± SD), that of protein 34 ± 11 g/day, and that of calcium 400 ± 250 mg/day. Our dietary survey confirms that elderly patients in hospital only eat part of their meals at best (23). In this group of patients with femoral neck fractures, the energy intake during hospital stay was inadequate, with a mean value corresponding to about 60% of the recommended allowance for elderly people: energy 1,800 kcal/day, protein 60 g/day, and calcium 1,000 mg/day (27,28). The spontaneous food intake can therefore be expected to perpetuate malnutrition, as previously reported in this type of patient (23,24).

Effects of Dietary Supplementation

The dietary supplementation increased the intake of energy by 23%, of protein by 62%, and of calcium by 130%. Given at 8 PM, the supplement did not interfere with the scheduled meals and thus did not reduce the voluntary oral intake. The oral protein-rich nutritional supplement given daily increased the energy intake close to the recommended allowances. Its ingestion was associated with biochemical evidence of nutritional improvement, as assessed by the serum albumin levels, which showed a significant increase in the supplemented patients. Such an improvement was obtained previously by using either nasogastric tube feeding or parenteral nutrition (24,25). Our study demonstrated that it can be achieved by providing a simple oral dietary preparation. This simplicity has some obvious practical and psychological advantages.

The clinical follow-up was significantly better in the supplemented group, with 56% having a favorable clinical outcome as compared to 13% in the control group ($p < 0.05$) during their stay in the convalescent hospital. The rate of complications and deaths were significantly ($p < 0.05$) lower in the supplemented (44%) than in the control group (87%). Six months after the fracture, the rate of complications and mortality remained significantly lower ($p < 0.02$) in supplemented patients (40%) than in controls (74%). Similarly, the median duration of the overall hospital stay was significantly shorter ($p < 0.02$) in the supplemented group (24 days) than in the patients receiving dietary supplement (40 days). Although the mean duration of the dietary supplementation did not exceed one month, the significantly lower rate of complications and deaths was still observed at 6 months. When mortality is considered alone, no patient belonging to the supplemented group died between the discharge day from the second hospital and the 6-month control as compared to six fatal outcomes in the control group. Again, these results are in good agreement with two previous studies made in patients with femoral neck fractures receiving dietary supplementation provided either by nasogastric tube or intravenous infusion (24,25). In both trials improvement in anthropometric variables and clinical outcome was documented (24,25). In our study, the differences in the biochemical and clinical evolution between the two groups of patients suggest that the nutritional state was rapidly influenced by the oral supplementation, while its clinical benefit became clearly apparent only after the acute traumatic phase (fracture, operation, and early postoperative days) was passed.

The results of this first controlled study suggested that the clinical outcome of elderly patients with femoral neck fracture can be improved by a simple oral dietary supplementation. Among the various nutritional elements that could have played a role, an inadequate protein intake might have been particularly important for the risk of hip fracture.

ROLE OF PROTEIN IN THE BENEFITS
OF DIETARY SUPPLEMENTATION

The major aim of this second prospective controlled study was to assess the clinical outcome of hip-fractured elderly patients receiving two different oral dietary supplements, which essentially differed by the presence or absence of protein. In addition, we also determined bone mineral density by dual photon absorptiometry (17) and followed its course at the lumbar spine, femoral neck, and femoral shaft levels in the two groups of patients.

Patients and Protein Supplementation

Sixty-two patients (mean age 82 years) admitted into the orthopedic ward for fracture of the proximal femur were randomized into two groups. One group comprised 33 patients aged 83.2 ± 1.3 years, who received 250 ml of an oral nutritional supplement containing protein (20.4 g), mineral salts (Ca 0.525 g), and vitamins (A = 750 IU; D_3 = 25 IU) daily for a mean of 38 days. A control group comprised 29 patients aged 81.3 ± 1.6 years and received 250 ml of an oral nutritional supplement containing the same amount of mineral salts and vitamins but no protein, for the same period of time. The evaluation of clinical outcome was based on the frequency of complications during the stay in both the orthopedic ward and the recovery hospital, as well as 7 months later.

Effects of Protein Supplementation

The clinical course was significantly better in the group receiving the protein-containing supplement, with 79% having a favorable course as compared to 36% ($p < 0.02$) in the control group during the stay in the recovery hospital. The rate of complications and deaths was also significantly lower in the protein-supplemented than in the control group (52% *vs.* 80%, $p < 0.05$) 7 months after hip fracture. The median duration of the hospital stay was significantly lower in the protein-supplemented group (69 *vs.* 102 days, $p < 0.05$). The present prospective randomized controlled investigation does not support the suggestion (29) that vitamin A could be the key nutritional element responsible for the favorable clinical outcome observed in the trial described above. The protein supplement provided a more than 60% increase in the overall daily protein consumption, taking into account that the supplement did not reduce the voluntary food intake. It should be stressed that the oral supplement increased the overall protein intake from a low to a normal level. A protein supplementation above the recommended allowance should be avoided since it may lead to a negative calcium balance (30–32).

Bone Mineral Density

On admission, both femoral neck and femoral shaft bone mineral density values were significantly lower in both groups as compared with age- and sex-matched healthy controls. Seven months after the fracture, no significant difference in bone mineral density between the protein-supplemented patients and the controls could be detected. However, the number of patients showing a significant decrease in femoral shaft density was significantly lower in the protein-supplemented group. This difference in bone density was associated with a greater increase in the plasma level of osteocalcin, taken as a reflection of osteoblastic activity.

CONCLUSION

A recent epidemiological survey emphasizes the high incidence, the dramatic consequences, and the important costs of osteoporotic fractures of the proximal femur in the Geneva region. Anthropometric and biochemical assessments confirm that elderly patients with hip fracture are often malnourished on admission. This malnutrition or undernutrition is more severe than that observed among the general elderly population. Bone mass measurement indicates that both women and men with hip fractures have a decreased mineral density at various sites of the skeleton. However, the difference appeared to be of higher magnitude for the femoral neck, suggesting a preferential bone loss at this site. Dietary survey indicates that nutritional requirements were not spontaneously met while the patients were in hospital, although adequate quantities of food were offered. In patients receiving a daily oral nutrition supplement for a mean period of 32 days (250 ml, 20 g protein, 254 kcal, 525 mg calcium, and various vitamins and minerals), the clinical outcome was significantly better, with reduction in both complication rate and median duration of hospital stay. The clinical benefits of this daily supplement appear to be essentially due to the increase in the protein intake as demonstrated in a prospective controlled randomized study where the effects of two dietary supplements that essentially differed by their protein content were compared. Finally, follow-up of bone mineral density suggests that normalization of the protein intake could prevent bone loss in undernourished elderly people after hip fracture, at least at the level of weight-bearing cortical bone. Further prospective studies are needed to confirm the possible benefit of protein supplementation to bone mass in undernourished elderly subjects.

ACKNOWLEDGMENTS

Studies described in this chapter were supported in part by the Swiss National Foundation (grant No 3200.025.535). We thank Dr. J.-M. Kahn (Sandoz Nutrition LTD) for supplying the nutritional supplements. The authors also wish to express their appreciation to Mrs. M.-C. Brandt for her secretarial assistance. R. Rizzoli is the recipient of a Max Cloetta career development award.

REFERENCES

1. Fenton Lewis A. Fracture of the neck of the femur: changing incidence. *Br Med J* 1981;283: 1217–9.
2. Boyce WJ, Vessey MP. Rising incidence of fracture of the proximal femur. *Lancet* 1985;i:150–1.
3. Nagant de Deuxchaisnes C, Devogelaer J-P. Increase in the incidence of hip fractures and the ratio of trochanteric to cervical hip fractures in Belgium. *Calcif Tissue Int* 1988;42:201–3.
4. Falch JA, Ilebekk A, Slungaard U. Epidemiology of hip fractures in Norway. *Acta Orthop Scand* 1985;56:12–6.
5. Melton LJ, III, O'Fallon WM, Riggs BL. Secular trends in the incidence of hip fractures. *Calcif Tissue Int* 1987;41:57–64.
6. Wallace WA. The increasing incidence of fractures of the proximal femur: an orthopaedic epidemic. *Lancet* 1983;i:1413–4.
7. Nydegger V, Rizzoli R, Rapin CH, Vasey H, Bonjour J-P. Incidence of fracture of proximal femur in Geneva (Switzerland) inhabitants. In: Christiansen C, Overgaard K, eds. *Osteoporosis 1990.* Copenhagen: Osteopress, 1990:182–3.
8. Tinetti ME, Speechley M, Ginter SF. Risks factors for falls among elderly persons living in the community. *N Engl J Med* 1988;319:1701–7.
9. Aniansson A, Zetterberg C, Hedberg M, Henriksson K. Impaired muscle function with aging. *Clin Orthop* 1984;191:193–201.
10. Dalen N, Hellström L-G, Jacobson B. Bone mineral content and mechanical strength of the femoral neck. *Acta Orthop Scand* 1976;47:503–8.
11. Esses SI, Lotz JC, Hayes WC. Biomechanical properties of the proximal femur determined in vitro by single-energy quantitative computed tomography. *J Bone Miner Res* 1989;4:715–22.
12. Riggs BL, Melton LJ. Involutional osteoporosis. *N Engl J Med* 1986;314:1676–86.
13. Cummings SR. Are patients with hip fractures more osteoporotic? *Am J Med* 1985;78:487–94.
14. Eriksson SA, Widhe TC. Bone mass in women with hip fracture. *Acta Orthop Scand* 1988;59: 19–23.
15. Mazess RB, Barden H, Ettinger M, Schultz E. Bone density of the radius, spine and proximal femur in osteoporosis. *J Bone Miner Res* 1988;3:13–18.
16. Chapuy MC, Duboeuf F, Haond P, Braillon P, Delmas PD, Meunier PJ. *Bone mineral density of the proximal femur measured by X-ray absorptiometry in elderly women with and without hip fractures.* Copenhagen: Abstract book of the Third International Symposium of Osteoporosis, 1990:76.
17. Slosman DO, Rizzoli R, Buchs B, Piana F, Donath A, Bonjour JP. Comparative study of the performance of X ray and Gd-153 bone densitometers at the levels of the spine, the femoral neck and the femoral shaft. *Eur J Nucl Med* 1990;17:3–9.
18. Chevalley T, Rizzoli R, Nydegger V, *et al.* Preferential low bone mineral density of the femoral neck in patients with a recent fracture of the proximal femur. *Osteoporosis Int* 1991;1:147–54.
19. Jensen JE, Jensen TG, Smith TK, Johnston DA, Dudrick SJ. Nutrition in orthopaedic surgery. *J Bone Joint Surg* 1982;64:1263–72.
20. Bruyère A, Rapin C-H, Dirren H. Nutritional blood values in patients with femoral neck fracture. A comparative study. In: Chandra RK, ed. *Nutrition, immunity and illness in the elderly.* London: Pergamon Press, 1984:242–6.
21. Wootton R, Brereton PJ, Clark MB, *et al.* Fractured neck of the femur in the elderly: an attempt to identify patients at risk. *Clin Sci* 1979;57:93–101.
22. Young GA, Chem C, Hill GL. Assessment of protein-caloric malnutrition in surgical patients from plasma proteins and anthropometric measurements. *Am J Clin Nutr* 1978;31:429–35.

23. Bastow MD, Rawkings J, Allison SP. Undernutrition, hypothermia, and injury in elderly women with fractured femur: an injury response to altered metabolism? *Lancet* 1983;1:143–6.
24. Bastow MD, Rawlings J, Allison SP. Benefits of supplementary tube feeding after fractured neck of femur: a randomized controlled trial. *Br Med J* 1983;287:1589–92.
25. Giaccaglia G, Malagù U, Antonelli M, Boschi S, Tabarroni I. Il supporto nutrizionale negli interventi di fratture dell'anca nell'anziano. Esperienze et risultati. *Minerva Anestesiol* 1986;52:397–400.
26. Delmi M, Rapin CH, Bengoa JM, Delmas PD, Vasey H, Bonjour JP. Dietary supplementation in elderly patients with fractured neck of the femur. *Lancet* 1990;i:1013–6.
27. FAO-OMS. *Manuel des besoins nutritionnels de l'homme.* Geneva: WHO, 1974:21–8.
28. National Research Council. Food and Nutrition Board. *Recommended dietary allowances.* Washington, DC: National Academy of Sciences, 1980.
29. Thurnham DI. Nutrition and hip fracture. *Lancet* 1990;335:1341–2.
30. Parfitt AM. Dietary risk factors for age-related bone loss and fractures. *Lancet* 1983;ii:1181–4.
31. Schaafsma G, Van Beresteyn ECH, Raymakers JA, Duursma SA. Nutritional aspects of osteoporosis. *World Rev Nutr Diet* 1987;49:121–59.
32. Yuen DE, Draper HH. Long-term effects of excess protein and phosphorus on bone homeostasis in adult mice. *J Nutr* 1983;113:1374–80.

DISCUSSION

This chapter was part of the Round-Table Conference on the prevention of osteoporosis. Please refer to the round-table discussion, page 187.

Nutrition of the Elderly, edited by H. Munro, and
G. Schlierf, Nestlé Nutrition Workshop Series, Vol. 29,
Nestec Ltd., Vevey/Raven Press, Ltd., New York © 1992.

The Effect of Estrogens in Prevention and Treatment of Osteoporosis

Robert Lindsay

*Regional Bone Center, Helen Hayes Hospital,
West Haverstraw, New York 10993, USA*

Osteoporosis is a disorder of the skeleton characterized by reduction in skeletal mass and a consequent alteration in architecture that increases the risk of fracture (1). The disorder is most evident among postmenopausal women, as Albright pointed out more than 50 years ago (2). In many countries osteoporosis has now been recognized as a major public health problem. It has been estimated that in the United States there result some 1.5 million fractures each year at a cost of $10 to $20 billion (3). An increase in the number of fractures is occurring as the population ages, and in some countries there appears to be an increase in age-specific incidence of the disorder, for reasons that are unknown.

PATHOPHYSIOLOGY

The amount of bone in the skeleton in the young adult is primarily under genetic control, but may be modified during growth by diet and physical activity. Peak bone mass, as this is called, is greater in men than in women (4). In addition, women begin to lose bone tissue as they approach menopause, or if ovarian failure occurs for any other reason (5). Thus, bone loss with age is ubiquitous among the female of the human species. The rate of loss of bone is greatest in areas of cancellous bone, the spongy bone that forms the center of vertebral bodies, and also occurs at other sites such as within the femoral neck. It is not surprising, therefore, that the most frequent fractures are those of the spine (so-called crush fractures) and hip, although fracture of any bone can occur (3).

Bone mass after menopause therefore depends on initial bone mass and rate of loss. Bone loss, while primarily occurring because of reduction in the supply of ovarian sex steroids, can be modified by a wide variety of other factors, often called risk factors. The most commonly cited risk factors are listed in Table 1.

Nutritional status contributes to skeletal status in several ways, but does not appear to influence significantly the rate of bone loss in the period immediately after menopause (6). Reduced calcium intake can clearly cause bone loss, principally by

TABLE 1. *Proposed risk factors for osteoporosis*

Genetic	High sodium
Race	High animal protein
Sex	**Lifestyle**
Familial prevalence	Cigarette use
Nutritional	Low physical activity
Low calcium intake	**Endocrine**
High alcohol	Menopausal age (oophorectomy)
High caffeine	Obesity

necessitating the use of skeletal calcium to maintain serum calcium constant in the presence of inadequate dietary supply. In the immediate phase after menopause, release of calcium from the skeleton is increased as estrogen levels decline, thereby allowing serum calcium to be sustained even when calcium intake is quite low. Consequently, calcium supplementation does not significantly reduce bone loss at this time of life, especially at sites of cancellous bone. A diet deficient in calcium is generally poor in other nutrients (RP Heaney, personal communication). Several nutritional abnormalities may also interfere in a negative way with skeletal homeostasis, including anorexia and bulimia as well as excess caffeine, alcohol, and possibly protein intake.

Gradual decline in physical activity with increasing age is also a contributor to bone loss. The skeleton can be considered to have a "mechanostat" that responds to the level of use (7). Thus, increasing use results in increments of skeletal mass. The converse is also true. One other lifestyle factor that may affect the skeleton is cigarette consumption, although the importance of this is not entirely clear.

In addition to nutritional and lifestyle factors, there are a variety of sporadic factors including excess thyroid hormone, glucocorticoid use, or excess endogenous production that can negatively affect the skeleton. The effects of all these risk factors are likely to be additive and cumulative in any individual, but cannot be used to assess accurately risk or skeletal status in the individual patient.

The availability of non-invasive techniques for measurement of bone mass has improved the capacity to estimate individual risk (8). Low bone mass is the single most important risk factor for fracture. Recent data have shown that low bone mass predicts not only future bone mass but also the risk of future fracture (8). Thus, a single estimate of bone mass can be used as a guide to determine those requiring preventive therapy.

PREVENTION

It is perhaps not surprising that if loss of ovarian hormones increases the rate of bone turnover and loss of skeletal tissue, replacement of those hormones reverses this effect (5,9). Many studies have now shown that estrogen intervention reduces the rate of bone loss in either postmenopausal women or ovariectomized women.

The effects can be seen immediately after loss of ovarian function and at least up to the age of 75 years (10) and in patients with established osteoporosis. The action of estrogen in slowing bone loss continues for as long as therapy is continued, and when treatment is stopped there is a corresponding increase in bone remodeling and bone loss begins again (11). The skeleton is extremely sensitive to the effects of estrogen and dose levels that supply sufficient estradiol to achieve mid-follicular serum levels appear to be capable of slowing bone loss. For conjugated equine estrogens, two studies have demonstrated that the minimum effective dose is 0.625 mg and that there is no advantage to increasing the dose further (12,13). The skeleton does not appear to be concerned about the route of administration, only the adequacy of the supplied dose, and estrogens given by any route that have been tested slow bone loss if adequate circulating concentrations can be achieved.

Long-term estrogen use, at least more than 5 years, is associated with a reduction in the risk of fractures of the hip and distal radius (5,14). Data also indicate that estrogens reduce the risk of vertebral crush fracture, possibly by as much as 75% (15,16). Thus, estrogen therapy would be expected to reduce significantly the impact of osteoporotic fractures among the aging female population. It is still not clear if these effects will persist after treatment is discontinued and it may be that to obtain maximum benefit, long-term, if not lifetime, therapy will be required.

Certain progestins also reduce bone turnover and the rate of bone loss. Those most commonly found to be effective belong to the class of progestins derived from 19-nortestosterone, and may be related to their androgenic or anabolic effects rather than to progestin activity (17). In most studies, the addition of a progestin to estrogen, used to protect the endometrium from long-term continuous exposure to estrogens, does not significantly influence the effect of estrogen on the skeleton. Recently, one study suggested that the addition of 1 mg per day norethindrone to an estrogen results in a more positive bone balance than could be achieved by estrogen alone (18). This study requires to be confirmed.

Other potential interactions of estrogen include those with the nutritional and lifestyle risk factors. One study suggests that the required estrogen dose can be reduced in the presence of a moderately high calcium intake of 1,500 mg/day (19). Another study indicates that the effects of estrogen on bone mass are greater when coupled with a resistance exercise program (20). Finally, published data suggest that estrogen metabolism may be altered by cigarette consumption to a degree that negatively affects the skeletal response (21). All of those data require further study.

Side Effects of Estrogen

The long-term exposure to estrogen significantly increases the risk of endometrial carcinoma (22). Daily doses of 0.625 mg of conjugated equine estrogen at least double the risk (an increase from 1:1,000 patient years to 2:1,000), whereas doubling the daily dose increases the risk from 4 to 8 times over baseline. The addition of a progestin reverses this effect. Progestins are most commonly provided in sequential fashion with 12 to 14 days of treatment each month. Our usual regimen is daily estrogen, 0.625 mg conjugated equine estrogen, on a continuous basis and medroxy-progesterone acetate 5 to 10 mg/day from day 1 through day 14 of each calendar month. This regimen results in monthly vaginal bleeding that is usually somewhat lighter than a regular period. If breast tenderness is a problem, estrogen can be omitted from day 14 of each month for 3 to 7 days. For those who prefer to avoid bleeding, if the patient is more than 3 years from menopause, a regimen of continuous therapy can be attempted (23). The usual is a combination of 0.625 mg conjugated equine estrogen in combination with medroxyprogesterone acetate 2.5 mg per day. In about 60% of cases or more vaginal bleeding ceases within 6 months and does not recur. The long-term safety of this regimen has yet to be tested adequately.

The most serious potential side effect of hormone therapy of postmenopausal women is the chance of an increase in the risk of breast cancer (24). The data are extremely mixed. Recent attempts at meta-analysis of the studies available suggest a small (10–20%) increase in risk associated with long-term therapy (>10 years) (25). The effect of the added progestin is not clear, and progestin may further increase the risk. For that reason, among others, progestins should not be used in the absence of a uterus. Since breast cancer is very common, there is good reason for ensuring that every postmenopausal woman have an annual mammography. There are no studies that indicate an increase in the mortality from breast cancer with estrogen use. There is a small but significant increase in the risk of gallstones associated with oral estrogen administration.

Estrogen administration to postmenopausal women appears to reduce the risk of ischemic heart disease significantly (26). Several epidemiological studies have examined this in detail. The general conclusion appears to be that long-term estrogen use is associated with a reduction in risk of about 50%, an extraordinary rate of protection if indeed it is accurate. There are potential mechanisms of action for this effect of estrogen. First, there is a clear increase in low-density lipoprotein across the menopause, an effect that is reversed by estrogen. Additionally, oral estrogens increase the circulating concentration of high-density lipoprotein (27). These are considered to be beneficial effects on lipoprotein metabolism, which might at least in part account for the effects on cardiac disease. In addition, estrogens are known to have receptors in arterial walls, and the physiological responses of coronary arteries are dependent on estrogen status (28). Vasodilator responses to physiological stimuli are changes to vasoconstrictor responses in the absence of estrogen, in animal models of coronary disease. Reduction in risk of cardiovascular disease will clearly outweigh all other effects of postmenopausal estrogen. The effect of added progestin is still not clear since progestins at least to some extent reverse the effects of estrogen on lipoprotein metabolism. One epidemiological study suggests that progestins do not significantly alter the estrogen effects, but clearly confirmatory studies are required.

Mode of Action of Estrogen

The mode of action of estrogen on the skeleton remains obscure. Recently, estrogen receptors have been found in cells of the osteoblast lineage (29). A variety of physiological responses have been described *in vitro* in response to incubation with biologically appropriate concentrations of estrogen. These include alteration in cell division, increased expression of the RNA of a variety of proteins known to be synthesized by osteoblasts including type 1 collagen, alkaline phosphatase, TGF-β, IGF-1, and osteocalcin. Others have been unable to detect significant responses in osteoblast-like cells unless transfected with estrogen receptors. Recently, one study could find no effects on primary cultures of human osteoblasts (30). Alternative actions of estrogens include the potential for steroids to mediate their effects on skeletal metabolism by affecting cells within marrow not normally considered to be directly involved in skeletal remodeling. Alterations in mast cell activity, or production of interleukins by cells of the monocyte macrophage series, are potential mechanisms for estrogens to affect skeletal homeostasis. Further studies of the direct effects of estrogens are required.

Estrogens could also modify skeletal remodeling by interacting with calcium homeostasis. Recently, we demonstrated that estrogens altered parathyroid sensitivity and increased the hydroxylation of 25-hydroxyvitamin D to its active metabolite 1,25-dihydroxyvitamin D. Increased production of this metabolite could account for the improved intestinal calcium absorption observed after estrogen administration (31). In part at least this may also explain the improved efficiency in utilization of nutritional calcium and thus the reduced calcium requirement to maintain calcium homeostasis, which appears to be about 1,000 mg/day, or 500 mg less than the daily requirement of estrogen-depleted women.

Alternatives to Estrogen

Alternatives to estrogen for prevention of bone loss are limited. Salmon calcitonin given either by subcutaneous or intranasal route can slow bone loss in the immediate postmenopausal period (32). Alterations in nutrition or physical activity cannot slow bone loss, but may potentially modify individual response to estrogen and must be considered when estrogens are used. There are limited data that suggest that bisphosphonates may also prevent bone loss, but insufficient data are available about the long-term effects of these medications for them to be recommended for use as preventive therapy.

Treatment of the established condition (i.e., after fracture has resulted in presentation of the patient to the clinician) allows the clinician limited choices. Estrogens are again first-line therapy. Calcitonin is an alternative, and potentially bisphosphonates can also be used. All of those agents, although acting through different mechanisms, reduce bone remodeling. Therefore, these agents are most likely to be effective in situations of increased turnover. When patients present after fracture, bone remodeling is only increased in the minority. However, in general most individuals appear to do relatively well when estrogens or calcitonin are used, although some data suggest that the response is somewhat better when high turnover can be documented. As yet there are no agents that increase bone formation and reliably reduce the risk of recurrent fracture, and the disorder is more easily prevented than treated.

CONCLUSION

Estrogen loss at the time of menopause (or at any time of life) increases skeletal remodeling and accelerates bone loss. Estrogen replacement prevents this process and reduces the risk of future fracture. The effects of estrogen in this regard are specific. Alteration in nutrition or physical activity cannot replace the effects of estrogen in the immediate years after menopause, but potentially may modify individual response to estrogen. Estrogens can also be used in treatment of the established disease. In addition to their effect on bone, estrogens also appear to reduce the risk of cardiovascular disease among postmenopausal women, but may increase the risk of breast cancer after prolonged use. Estrogen use is associated with an overall reduction in mortality among postmenopausal women.

ACKNOWLEDGMENTS

Supported by grant numbers AR 39191 and DK 42892 from the National Institutes of Health.

REFERENCES

1. Consensus Development Conference. Osteoporosis. *Am J Med* 1991;90:107–10.
2. Albright F, Smith PH, Richardson AM. Postmenopausal osteoporosis. *JAMA* 1941;116:2465–74.
3. Melton LJ III. Epidemiology of fractures. In: Riggs BL, ed. *Osteoporosis: etiology, diagnosis and management.* New York: Raven Press, 1988:133–54.
4. Garn SM, Nagy JM, Sandusky ST. Differential sexual dimorphism in bone parameters of subjects of European and African ancestry. *Am J Phys Anthropol* 1972;37:127–30.
5. Lindsay R. Sex steroids in the pathogenesis and prevention of osteoporosis. In: Riggs BL, ed. *Osteoporosis: etiology, diagnosis and management.* New York: Raven Press, 1988:333–58.
6. Dawson-Hughes B, Dallal GE, Krall EA, Sadowski L, Sahyoun N, Tannenbaum S. A controlled trial of the effect of calcium supplementation on bone density in postmenopausal women. *N Engl J Med* 1990;323:878–83.
7. Frost HM. The pathomechanics of osteoporosis. *Clin Orthop Rel Res* 1986;200:198–225.
8. Johnston CC, Melton LJ, III, Lindsay R, Eddy DM. Clinical indications for bone mass measurement. *J Bone Miner Res* 1989;4(suppl):1–28.
9. Lindsay R. Osteoporosis and its relationship to estrogen. *Contemp Obstet Gynecol* 1984;63:201–24.
10. Lindsay R, Tohme J. Estrogen treatment of patients with established postmenopausal osteoporosis. *Obstet Gynecol* 1990;76:1–6.
11. Lindsay R, Hart DM, MacLean A, Clark AC, Kraszewski A, Garwood J. Bone response to termination of oestrogen treatment. *Lancet* 1978;i:1325–7.
12. Lindsay R, Hart DM, Clark DM. The minimum effective dose of estrogen for prevention of postmenopausal bone loss. *Obstet Gynecol* 1984;63:759–63.
13. Genant HK, Cann CE, Ettinger B, Gordon GS. Quantitative computed tomography of vertebral spongiosa: a sensitive method for detecting early bone loss after oophorectomy. *Ann Intern Med* 1982;97:699–705.
14. Weiss NS, Ure CL, Ballard JH. Decreased risk of fractures of the hip and lower forearm with postmenopausal use of oestrogen. *N Engl J Med* 1980;303:1195–8.

15. Lindsay R, Hart DM, Forrest C, Baird C. Prevention of spinal osteoporosis in oophorectomized women. *Lancet* 1980;ii:1151–4.
16. Ettinger B, Genant HK, Cann CE. Long-term estrogen therapy prevents bone loss and fracture. *Ann Intern Med* 1985;102:319–24.
17. Abdalla HI, Hart DM, Lindsay R, Leggate I, Hooke A. Prevention of bone mineral loss in post-menopausal women by norethisterone. *Obstet Gynecol* 1985;66:789–92.
18. Christiansen C, Riis BJ. Beta-estradiol and continuous norethisterone: a unique treatment for established osteoporosis in elderly women. *J Clin Endocrinol Metab* 1990;71:836–41.
19. Ettinger B, Genant HK, Cann CE. Postmenopausal bone loss is prevented by treatment with low-dosage estrogen with calcium. *Ann Intern Med* 1987;106:40–5.
20. Notelovitz M, Martin D, Tesar R, *et al.* Estrogen therapy and variable resistance weight training increases bone mineral in surgically menopausal women. *J Bone Miner Res* 1991;6:583–90.
21. Christiansen C, Riis BJ. 17 Beta-estradiol and continuous norethisterone: a unique treatment for established osteoporosis in elderly women. *J Clin Endocrinol Metab* 1990;71:836–41.
22. Mack TM, Pike MC, Henderson BE, *et al.* Estrogens and endometrial cancer in a retirement community. *N Engl J Med* 1976;294:1262–7.
23. Clisham PR, de Zeigler D, Lozano K, Judd HL. Comparison of continuous versus sequential estrogen and progestin therapy in postmenopausal women. *Obstet Gynecol* 1991;77:241–6.
24. Bergkvist L, Adami HO, Persson I, Hoover R, Schairer C. The risk of breast cancer after estrogen and estrogen-progestin replacement. *N Engl J Med* 1989;321:293–7.
25. Dupont WD, Page DL. Menopausal estrogen replacement therapy and breast cancer. *Arch Intern Med* 1991;151:67–72.
26. Ross RK, Paganini-Hill A, Mack TM. Menopausal oestrogen therapy and protection from death from ischemic heart disease. *Lancet* 1981;i:858–60.
27. Notelovitz M, Gudat SC, Ware MD, Dougherty MC. Oestrogen-progestin therapy and the lipid balance of postmenopausal women. *Maturitas* 1985;7:141–6.
28. Clarkson TB, Shivley CA, Morgan TM, Koritnik DR, Adams MR, Kaplan JR. Oral contraceptives and coronary artery atherosclerosis of cynomolgus monkeys. *Obstet Gynecol* 1990;75:217–22.
29. Erikssen EF, Colvard DS, Berg NJ. Evidence of estrogen receptors in normal human osteoblast-like cells. *Science* 1988;241:84–6.
30. Keeting PE, Scott RE, Colvard DS, Han IK, Spelsberg TC, Riggs BL. Lack of a direct effect on proliferation and differentiation of normal human osteoblast-like cells. *J Bone Miner Res* 1991;6:297–304.
31. Cosman F, Shen V, Herrington BS, Seibel M, Ratcliffe A, Lindsay R. Mechanism of estrogen action in osteoporosis treatments as assessed by human (1-34)PTH infusion. In: Overgaard K, Christiansen C, eds. *Osteoporosis.* Copenhagen: Osteopress, 1990:976–8.
32. Reginster JY, Albert A, Lecart MP, *et al.* 1-Year controlled randomized trial of prevention of early postmenopausal bone loss by intranasal calcitonin. *Lancet* 1987;ii:1481–3.

DISCUSSION

This chapter was part of the Round-Table Conference on prevention of osteoporosis. Please refer to the round-table discussion, page 187.

Nutrition of the Elderly, edited by H. Munro, and
G. Schlierf, Nestlé Nutrition Workshop Series, Vol. 29,
Nestec Ltd., Vevey/Raven Press, Ltd., New York © 1992.

Exercise in the Prevention of Osteoporosis

Carol N. Meredith

*Division of Clinical Nutrition, School of Medicine, University of California at Davis,
Davis, California 95616, USA*

Osteoporosis is a weakening of the skeleton due to a decrease in mineral content and a change in bone architecture. It continues to be an incurable, debilitating, and painful condition of the elderly, especially women. The cost to the United States is $10–20 billion dollars a year, and is likely to increase as more persons live to advanced old age.

Bone loss occurs throughout adult life. Bones are continually being remodeled, and the slight inefficiencies of bone turnover result in a gradual loss of mineral, especially from trabecular bone. Persons who begin their adult life with a large bone mass may never suffer from osteoporosis because their bone density will not fall below the fracture threshold. The first step in preventing osteoporosis is ensuring that children and adolescents acquire the largest possible bone mass consistent with their genetic possibilities. High peak bone mass is mainly an inherited trait, but the intake of calcium and other nutrients, endocrine status, and exercise habits also affect bone acquisition. Some 60% of peak bone mass is acquired during adolescence, making this a period of vulnerability to low calcium intake and endocrine changes that impair adequate development. As physical activity and diet can usually be modified at will, these interventions during adolescence, the adult years, and old age have been the subject of much research.

Physical activity covers a very broad range. Persons can be almost completely inactive (e.g., patients with severe arthritis, or with neuromuscular diseases) or so athletic that they require more than 5,000 kcal/day to maintain body weight. Clearly, bone density is different for these two extremes. Most persons in developed countries lead quite sedentary lives, spending nearly all of their time lying down, sitting, standing, or walking slowly. As they age, their physical activity declines further. What advice should they get about exercise that will prevent osteoporosis? From a public health point of view, we need to address the type and intensity of physical exercise that is appropriate for gaining and maintaining optimum bone mass throughout life. More recently, scientists are inquiring about the interactions between exercise and other treatments, such as increased calcium intake or hormone treatment, to determine their combined effect on bone health.

MECHANISMS UNDERLYING BONE MASS INCREASE WITH EXERCISE

In the last century, Wolff observed that bone was shaped according to the forces it sustained (1). If you compress or pull a bone to apply *stress* (force/cross-section), the bone undergoes *strain* (deformation/length). The trabecular density of a bone is the result of the sum of all loading events over time. Studies in experimental animals show that stress increases bone mineral, and that both the rate and total load have an effect. Intermittent stress is more effective than constant stress, but the total load applied is more important that the frequency of stress. The molecular basis for changes in bone architecture due to exercise is not known, nor is it possible to examine bone architecture *in vivo* and non-invasively. Studies in humans are based on measurements of bone mineral density, which predicts most but not all of the variability in bone strength.

The mechanism for translating stress/strain into increased bone mass is not well understood. One mechanism could be a local resistance to the resorbing effects of circulating parathyroid hormone, but the mediator is not known. As stress/strain acts locally, it has been suggested that the deformation of the elastic molecules in the matrix surrounding osteoblasts and osteoclasts imparts a message. Lanyon and his colleagues have suggested that proteoglycans in the bone may act as a messenger. These are highly charged molecules that can alter the electrochemical environment as they become more aligned. Loading applied as compression or torsion increases the alignment of proteoglycans in bone, to an extent that depends on the amount of applied strain (2). The increased orientation persists for some 48 hours, providing a local memory of loading to the system.

A fundamental cause of stress/strain on the skeleton is the weight of the body while standing, walking, or carrying out more vigorous activities. Obesity, with all its disadvantages, is actually protective of bone health. Hip fractures are more frequent among persons with lower body mass index (weight/height^2), lower body fat, and lower muscle mass (3). Persons who are overweight due to a large muscle mass or to obesity have denser and larger bones (4). In adolescent girls, body mass index is the best predictor of bone mineral density of the whole body (5). Totally taking away the stimulus of weight, such as during bed rest or microgravity, rapidly produces bone loss, in addition to other deconditioning effects (6). Weight-bearing, even if it is sporadic and not associated with exercise, can prevent the massive bone loss produced by bed rest (7). An hour of quiet standing every day in men otherwise confined to bed proved sufficient to conserve bone mineral (7). During convalescence from illness, or in severely deconditioned frail elderly people, rehabilitation activities that promote sitting, standing, and some walking may prevent accelerated bone loss.

Activities that provide intermittent but powerful compressive loads have a marked effect. This can be seen in the difference in radius width and mineral density between the dominant and non-dominant arm of tennis players (8). Activities that are not weight-bearing may also increase bone density by increasing the size, strength, and activity of muscles attached to bones. An analysis of cadavers found a linear relationship between the weight of the psoas muscles and the ash content of the vertebrae

(9). Similarly, there is a linear relationship between isometric strength of the back extensors and mineral density of the lumbar spine in older women (10). Although some studies have found increased bone mineral density of the spine in swimmers, the activities that most benefit bone health involve the load of body weight or extraneous weights.

EXERCISE AND THE ACCUMULATION OF PEAK BONE MASS

Exercise promotes linear growth in well-fed children (11), and therefore stimulates bone growth. This could be due to hormonal as well as paracrine or electrochemical effects on the skeleton.

Cross-sectional comparisons of sedentary or active young adults show differences of 10% to 40% in the bone density of various sites. Exercises that emphasize load may provide greater stress to the bones. A comparison of runners (high frequency, moderate load on the skeleton), weight-trained men (low frequency, very high load on the skeleton), and circuit-trained men (moderate frequency, high load on the skeleton) showed the highest values for the circuit-trained men, followed by the weight-trained group, and last the aerobically trained group (12). Exercise that promotes muscle growth and strength may favor increased bone density. Muscle strength is an independent predictor of bone mineral density, accounting for 15% to 20% of the variance in bone density of young women (13).

In college-age women, there is a linear relationship between the energy expended in exercise and vertebral bone mineral density in young normally menstruating women (14).

Exercise can affect bone health indirectly, through its effects on food intake and endocrine status. Young women gymnasts, dancers, runners, and ice skaters are encouraged to maintain a very lean physique. There are two consequences of this desire to lose weight. First, food intake is reduced, thus lowering the intake of calcium and other nutrients at a time of rapid skeletal growth. Second, the young woman's endocrine status may adapt, with a decline in reproductive hormones. There may be a delay in menarche, or a subsequent loss of menstrual cycles (amenorrhea). In women who begin a rigorous training program, amenorrhea is more likely if the diet is curtailed (15). Not all athletic women experience amenorrhea: it is more likely in those who are younger, vegetarian, thin, consume insufficient energy, and who have some sort of eating disorder (16). The loss of estrogen has dramatic effects on bone. Amenorrheic athletes have lower mineral density of the spine and the whole skeleton, compared to normally menstruating athletes or sedentary controls (Table 1). Bone strength is reduced, as shown by the greater incidence of stress fractures (20) and scoliosis (21). Studies of amenorrheic athletes in their twenties have shown that with a reduction in training intensity, menstrual cycles resume and there is an increase in vertebral bone mineral density (22). However, in young athletes, skeletal health is affected by poor bone accretion as well as by bone loss. In anorectic young girls, recovery of bone mass is a function of weight gain as well as recovery of normal

TABLE 1. *Lumbar bone mineral density in active young women: effects of amenorrhea*

	% of value for sedentary, normally menstruating women	
Reference	Amenorrheic	Eumenorrheic
(17)	89	108
(18)	91	110
(19)	85	98

menstrual status (23). Young women training for competition, who want to maintain low weight, may not accept a reduction in exercise activities or an increase in energy intake, in order to improve bone health. Increasing calcium intake alone will not improve their bone health (5), and endocrine treatments may be undesirable in young girls who have not yet reached adult height and body composition. The effects of strenuous training on endocrine status and bone health have not been as well studied in men.

Habitual physical exercise combined with a good diet is likely to favor bone health. When both calcium intake and exercise habits were examined in young women with normal menstrual cycles, active women consuming more than 800 mg/day of calcium had the highest lumbar bone mineral density, whereas sedentary women consuming less than 800 mg/day had the lowest values (14). These relationships may be less important in men, whose calcium intake is substantially higher than for women.

The problem with cross-sectional studies is that persons who already have superior muscles, bones, and motor coordination are more likely to become athletes. Intervention studies show less dramatic effects of exercise and often illustrate some of the disadvantages of training, such as injuries. In a 14-week study of a group of Israeli men undergoing military service, examined before and after extremely rigorous training, 40% of the men failed to complete the study, mostly because of stress injuries (24). They had to march, jog, and run, with and without heavy backpacks, for 8 hours a day, 6 days a week. Those completing the program showed an 11% increase in the bone mineral density of the left tibia, which is a remarkably high response for such a brief intervention. However, had these men been volunteers in an exercise program rather than army conscripts, another effect would have been a substantial dropout rate from the program.

EXERCISE AND THE PRESERVATION OF BONE

Many attempts have been made to slow the loss of bone that occurs in adult life, especially during and immediately after menopause. Estrogen replacement therapy has proved to be an effective treatment not only for delaying osteoporosis in women but also for preventing cardiovascular disease. Changes in diet and exercise also help preserve bone mass, and are worth pursuing because they improve health and well-being in a variety of ways.

TABLE 2. *Effects of weight-bearing exercise on the change in vertebral mineral density of women: longitudinal studies of 9 to 12 months*

Women	Reference	Exercise (%)	No exercise (%)
Postmenopausal	(28)	+2.5	−2.4
	(29)	+3.5	−2.7
	(30)	+4.9	−0.8
	(31)	+1.2	−6.0
	(32)	−5.6	−4.0
Premenopausal	(33)[a]	+0.8	−0.5

[a] Heavy resistance training.

Middle-aged men who have been active for 25 years or more have a higher bone mineral density than sedentary men (25). Women who take up running after menopause may provide divergent stimuli to their bones: increased stress/strain while running, but a decreased effect of mass if they lose body weight, and a lower capacity for producing bone-conserving steroidal hormones in their adipose tissue. Lumbar bone mineral density in lean middle-aged women runners was not different from the values for sedentary and heavier women (26).

Exercise intervention studies are effective. In 63-year-old women who had been losing 2% to 3% of bone mineral per year from the radius, a year of loading exercises for the arms produced a 3.8% gain in bone mineral (27). Weight-bearing aerobic exercise used in several studies has been shown, with few exceptions, to increase lumbar bone mineral density and the mineral density of other stressed sites. Some of these interventions in women are summarized in Table 2. The single study that showed no change with exercise involved less vigorous and prolonged activity (i.e., walking for a total of 120 minutes per week), no calcium supplements, and no estrogen treatment (32). In the study showing the most marked response, the women combined walking with some weight training, some were on estrogen therapy, and all were provided with a substantial calcium supplement of 1,500 mg/day (26). The benefits of exercise training are not permanent. After resuming sedentary habits, bone mineral density returns to baseline values (30).

The indirect effects of beginning an exercise program in older persons can help prevent some of the consequences of bone loss. Falling is usually the cause of bone fracture. Older persons who walk more than 3 miles (4.8 km) per week are less likely to suffer fractures (34). A review of six studies showed that muscle weakness, especially of the hip extensors, was a major risk factor for falling (35). Habitual exercise increases endurance, strength, coordination, and balance and thus improves the way persons negotiate hazards and take corrective action when they stumble or trip. In the elderly, the effort of walking, climbing stairs, and other everyday activities that help maintain bone mass becomes less strenuous after a certain amount of training. Physical activity, even if it is very mild, takes time away from hours of bone-losing activities such as lying down, lounging, or sitting. Physical activity demands energy, and active persons are likely to eat more food, making it easier for them to satisfy their needs for calcium, vitamin D, zinc, magnesium, and other nutrients that are important for the health of their musculoskeletal system.

CONCLUSION

Physical activity favors increased bone mineral density, especially if the diet provides adequate calcium and other nutrients. During growth, the most important way to improve bone health may be to increase the intake of dairy products. During and after menopause, estrogen treatment may be the most effective way to prevent bone loss. However, physical activity also has a role throughout life. In older women, exercise can prevent bone loss from certain sites. The changes are modest but significant. They disappear if the activity is not sustained. Excessive physical activity can be harmful; it can cause stress fractures and, in susceptible young women, lead to amenorrhea. Without normal menstrual cycles, thin and active young women develop osteopenia, increasing their risk of osteoporosis in old age. Habitual exercise is useful for ameliorating many conditions and diseases of older persons, such as diabetes mellitus or cardiovascular disease. It should also be advocated for improving bone health.

REFERENCES

1. Chanay A, Tschantz P. Mechanical influences in bone remodeling: experimental research on Wolff's law. *J Biomech* 1972;5:173–80.
2. Skerry TM, Suswillo R, El Haj AJ, Dodds RA, Lanyon LE. Load-induced proteoglycan orientation in bone tissue in vivo and in vitro. *Calcif Tissue Int* 1990;46:318–26.
3. Farmer ME, Harris T, Madans JH, Wallace RB, Cornoni-Huntley J, White LR. Anthropometric indicators and hip fracture. The NHANES I epidemiologic follow-up study. *J Am Geriatr Soc* 1989;37:9–16.
4. Liel Y, Edwards J, Shary J, Spicer KM, Gordon L, Bell NH. The effects of race and body habitus on bone mineral density of the radius, hip, and spine in premenopausal women. *J Clin Endocrinol Metab* 1988;66:1247–50.
5. Bachrach LK, Guido D, Katzman D, Litt IF, Marcus R. Decreased bone density in adolescent girls with anorexia nervosa. *Pediatrics* 1990;86:440–7.
6. Donaldson CK, Hulley SB, Vogel JM, Hattner RS, Bayers JH, McMillan DE. Effect of prolonged bed rest on bone mineral. *Metabolism* 1970;19:1071–84.
7. Issekutz B, Blizzard JJ, Birkhead NC, Rodahl K. Effect of prolonged bed rest on urinary calcium output. *J Appl Physiol* 1966;21:1013–20.
8. Jones HH, Priest JD, Hayes WC, Tichenon CC, Nagel DA. Humeral hypertrophy in response to exercise. *J Bone Joint Surg* 1977;59A:204–8.
9. Doyle F, Brown J, Lachance C. Relation between bone mass and muscle weight. *Lancet* 1970:i: 391–3.
10. Sinaki M, McPhee MC, Hodgson SF, Merritt JM, Offord KP. Relationship between bone mineral density of spine and strength of back extensors in healthy postmenopausal women. *Mayo Clin Proc* 1986;61:116–22.
11. Young VR, Torún B. Physical activity: impact on protein and amino acid metabolism and implications for nutritional requirements. In: *Nutrition in health and disease and international development.* New York: Alan R Liss, 1981:57–85.
12. Block JE, Genant HK, Black D. Greater vertebral bone mineral mass in exercising young men. *West J Med* 1986;145:39–42.

13. Snow-Harter C, Bouxsein M, Lewis B, Charette S, Weinstein P, Marcus R. Muscle strength as a predictor of bone mineral density in young women. *J Bone Miner Res* 1990;5:589–95.
14. Kanders B, Dempster DW, Lindsay R. Interaction of calcium nutrition and physical activity on bone mass in young women. *J Bone Miner Res* 1988;3:145–9.
15. Bullen BA, Skrinar GS, Beirins IZ, Von Mering G, Rurnbull BA, McArthur JW. Induction of menstrual disorders by strenuous exercise in untrained women. *N Engl J Med* 1985;312:1349–53.
16. Meredith CN, Dwyer JT. Nutrition and exercise: effects on adolescent health. *Annu Rev Public Health* 1991;12:309–33.
17. Drinkwater BL, Nilson K, Chesnut CH, Breamner WJ, Shainholtz S, Southworth MB. Bone mineral content of amenorrheic and eumenorrheic athletes. *N Engl J Med* 1984;311:277–81.
18. Marcus R, Cann C, Madvig P. Menstrual function and bone mass in elite women distance runners. *Ann Intern Med* 1985;102:158–63.
19. Nelson ME, Fisher EC, Catsos PD, Meredith CN, Turksoy RN, Evans WJ. Diet and bone status in amenorrheic athletes. *Am J Clin Nutr* 1986;43:910–6.
20. Barrow GW, Saha S. Menstrual irregularity and stress fractures in collegiate female distance runners. *Am J Sports Med* 1988;16:209–15.
21. Warren MP, Brooks-Gunn J, Hamilton LH, Warren LF, Hamilton WG. Scoliosis and fractures in young ballet dancers. *N Engl J Med* 1986;314:1348–53.
22. Drinkwater BL, Nilson K, Ott S, Chesnut CH. Bone mineral density after resumption of menses in amenorrheic athletes. *JAMA* 1986:256:380–2.
23. Bachrach LK, Katzman DK, Litt IF, Guido D, Marcus R. Recovery from osteopenia in adolescent girls with anorexia nervosa. *J Clin Endocrinol Metab* 1991;72:602–6.
24. Margulies JY, Simkin A, Leichter I, *et al*. Effect of intense physical activity on the bone-mineral content in the lower limbs of young adults. *J Bone Joint Surg* 1986;68:1090–3.
25. Dalén N, Olsson KE. Bone mineral content and physical activity. *Acta Orthop Scand* 1974;45:170–4.
26. Nelson ME, Meredith CN, Dawson-Hughes B, Evans WJ. Hormone and bone mineral status in endurance-trained and sedentary postmenopausal women. *J Clin Endocrinol Metab* 1988;66:927–33.
27. Ayalon J, Simkin A, Leichter I, Raifmann S. Dynamic bone loading exercises for postmenopausal women: effect on the density of the distal radius. *Arch Phys Med Rehabil* 1987;68:280–3.
28. Aloia JF, Cohn SH, Ostuni JA, Cane R, Ellis K. Prevention of involutional bone loss by exercise. *Ann Intern Med* 1978;89:356–8.
29. Krolner B, Toft B, Nielsen SP, Tondevold E. Physical exercise as prophylaxis against involutional vertebral bone loss: a controlled trial. *Clin Sci* 1983;64:541–6.
30. Dalsky GP, Stocke KS, Ehsani AA, Slatopolsky E, Lee WC, Birge SJ. Weight-bearing exercise training and lumbar bone mineral content in postmenopausal women. *Ann Intern Med* 1988;108:824–8.
31. Nelson ME, Fisher EC, Evans WJ. A one-year walking program and increased dietary calcium in postmenopausal women: effects on bone. *Am J Clin Nutr* 1991;53:1304–11.
32. Cavanaugh DJ, Cann CE. Brisk walking does not stop bone loss in postmenopausal women. *Bone* 1988;9:201–4.
33. Blake P, Protas EJ, Leblanc AD, Schneider VS, Evans HJ. Effects of weight lifting on bone mineral density in premenopausal women. *J Bone Miner Res* 1990;5:153–8.
34. Sorock GS, Bush TL, Golden AL, Fried LP, Breuer B, Hale WE. Physical activity and fracture risk in a free-living elderly cohort. *J Gerontol* 1988;43:134–9.
35. Robbins AS, Rubenstein LZ, Josephson KR, Schulman BL, Osterweil D, Fine G. Predictors of falls among elderly people. *Arch Intern Med* 1989;149:1628–33.

DISCUSSION

This chapter was part of the Round-Table Conference on prevention of osteoporosis. Please refer to the round-table discussion, page 187.

Nutrition of the Elderly, edited by H. Munro, and
G. Schlierf, Nestlé Nutrition Workshop Series, Vol. 29,
Nestec Ltd., Vevey/Raven Press, Ltd., New York © 1992.

Fluoride Therapy for Vertebral Osteoporosis

Pierre J. Meunier

*INSERM Unit 234, Edouard Herriot Hospital,
69437 Lyon, Cedex 3, France*

Vertebral osteoporosis is characterized by a predominant atrophy of spongy bone inducing non-traumatic vertebral fractures. Because a low bone mass is the major determinant of fracture risk, the ideal therapy for established vertebral osteoporosis should increase trabecular bone mass substantially, thereby decreasing the risk of new crush fractures. This ideal treatment should also be capable of restoring the normal architecture of bone in order to maintain its mechanical properties. Treatments acting by decreasing bone resorption can maintain existing bone mass or protect spongy bone architecture, but cannot substantially increase bone mass in order to decrease the occurrence of new vertebral fractures. Of the antiresorptive drugs, calcitonin has never been shown capable of reducing vertebral fracture rate in established osteoporosis, and the promising results recently obtained with an intermittent cyclical treatment with etidronate given for 2 years in osteoporosis (1) have not been confirmed by a follow-up of 346 patients during the third year of treatment with the drug.

In contrast, regimens that stimulate bone formation have the potential of increasing bone mass, and fluoride is one of the most effective of these regimens because of its ability to increase the osteoblast cell population. Fluoride was proposed as a curative therapy for vertebral crush fracture syndrome 30 years ago, and this idea was suggested by the massive increase in trabecular bone density of the axial skeleton that characterizes skeletal fluorosis radiologically and the low prevalence of osteoporosis in areas with moderately high fluoride concentrations in drinking water. Since 1961, several prospective open studies have shown that fluoride salts (sodium fluoride or monofluorophosphate) are effective in increasing trabecular bone mass. This was shown first by radiological techniques, then by histomorphometric analysis of iliac bone biopsies, and by measurements of the mineral bone density of the axial skeleton using dual photon absorptiometry, quantitative computed tomography, or neutron activation analysis. The stimulating effect on bone formation was confirmed by the increase in serum osteocalcin levels. These data led to a general agreement that sodium fluoride, combined with adequate calcium supplementation, has an anabolic effect on vertebral bone mass, and fluoride therapy has been approved for the treatment of established vertebral osteoporosis in nine European countries (Austria, Belgium, France, Germany, Ireland, Luxembourg, The Netherlands, Norway, and Switzerland) on the basis of studies using moderate or low doses of 15 to 25 mg/day of fluoride ion.

Uncertainties persisted, however, about the effectiveness of this treatment in decreasing the vertebral fracture rate, the effects on the risk of non-vertebral fractures related to the changes induced in cortical bone mass, the incidence of side effects limiting the clinical usefulness of fluoride treatment, especially gastrointestinal disorders and lower extremity pain syndrome. The statement published after the Consensus Development Conference held at Aalborg, October 3–4, 1987, concluded (2): "Fluoride may be used to increase trabecular bone mass in patients with severe vertebral osteoporosis. It is the only agent that has been shown to have a sustained effect on the formation of trabecular bone, both at appendicular and at axial sites. . . . Whether treatment with fluoride reduces the rate of vertebral fracture is not known. Prospective controlled studies now in place should help clarify this issue. . . . The optimum dose and duration of fluoride treatment are not known, but the duration should probably not exceed five years."

Four years after this statement, several new studies have been now achieved and it is possible to answer, at least in part, most of the questions raised in 1987. These recent advances consisted first of the results of two large clinical prospective controlled trials carried out in France (3) and in the United States (4), both of which analyzed the risk–benefit ratio of fluoride–calcium combined therapy in established vertebral osteoporosis. These two studies using different doses reached different conclusions and will be detailed below. In addition, the Proceedings of the International Workshop on Fluoride and Bone held at Niagara-on-the-Lake, October 12–15, 1988, and published as a supplement of the *Journal of Bone and Mineral Research* in March, 1990, included 32 papers emphasizing in particular the importance of both the dosage and the bioavailability of fluoride salt preparations (sodium fluoride and monofluorophosphate), discussing the effects of fluoride on bone tissue and bone cells and the mechanisms of fractures in osteoporotic patients treated with fluoride (5). Moreover, in these last 3 years several papers on fluoride have been published in specialized journals and many abstracts presented in large international conferences, including the 3rd International Symposium on Osteoporosis held in Copenhagen, October 14–20, 1990, and where more than 20 studies on fluoride have been discussed.

EFFICACY: INFLUENCE OF DOSE AND BIOAVAILABILITY ON THE CHANGES IN THE VERTEBRAL, FRACTURE RATE, AND IN BONE DENSITY

Table 1 summarizes the main characteristics of the target population and the main results from the French INSERM collaborative study (3), the Mayo Clinic study (4), and also the 4-year study carried out at the Henry Ford Hospital in Detroit (6) with the same daily dose of sodium fluoride (NaF) as the one given in the Mayo Clinic

TABLE 1. *Main characteristics and results of three recent controlled studies*

	Mamelle *et al.,* 1988 (3)	Riggs *et al.,* 1990 (4)	Kleerekoper *et al.,* 1990 (6)
Type of study	C (other therapies) P	C (1,500 mg Ca) P; DB	C (1,500 mg Ca) P; DB
Daily dose NaF (mg)	50 (Osteofluor 25)	90 day 1 60 day 2 mean: 75	75 (90–60)
Preparation	Enteric-coated tablets	Nonenteric coated capsules	Nonenteric coated capsules
No. patients enrolled	446	202	84
Duration of treatment (yrs)	2	4	4
Effect on vertebral fracture rate	Significant reduction (−25%)	Nonsignificant reduction (−15%)	Nonsignificant
Effect on nonvertebral complete fractures	Nonsignificant	Nonsignificant	Nonsignificant
Effect on lumbar bone mineral density	Not determined	+35% ($p < 0.0001$)	Not determined
Effect on radial shaft bone mineral content	Not determined	−4% ($p < 0.02$)	Not determined

C, controlled; P, prospective; DB, double blind.

study. The French study used a low dose (50 mg/day) of NaF given as enteric-coated tablets for 2 years and showed a significant reduction in vertebral fracture rate. The Mayo Clinic study used a higher dose (75 mg/day) of NaF given as nonenteric-coated capsules for 4 years. With this dose the authors noted that the number of new vertebral fractures over the whole study period was not different in the NaF group and the control group receiving calcium. It must be emphasized that the analysis of vertebral x-rays in the French study was performed blindly in only a quarter of the patients, selected at random. Riggs *et al.,* in a recent paper (4), questioned the results obtained in this study and suggested that the reduction in the vertebral fracture rate was not significant. After reanalysis of their data, the authors have confirmed that the 25% reduction in vertebral fractures after 2 years of treatment was significant, when calculated by the methods used by Riggs *et al.* (4). They calculated rates per person-year and found, between 0 and 24 months, 173 crush fractures per 360 patient years (rate: 0.48) in the NaF group, and 174 fractures per 272 patient year (rate: 0.64) in the non-NaF group. This 25% reduction is significant (chi square 15.8, $p < 0.001$).

The Mayo Clinic study has given rise to several recent comments, mainly calling into question the high mean daily dose (75 mg NaF), the preparation used (30 mg NaF nonenteric-coated capsules), and the duration of treatment (4 years) (8–10). In this study the daily fluoride ion dosage of 34 mg was 35% higher than the maximum dose of 25 mg recommended by the status report published after the Workshop on Fluoride and Bone held in Ontario, Canada, October 12–15, 1988 (11). Moreover, the bioavailability of NaF contained in the nonenteric-coated 30-mg capsules used in the Mayo Clinic study has been found much greater than that provided by enteric-coated tablets containing the same amount of NaF (10): the C max was found to be twice as high (21.3 *vs.* 10.1 μmol/L), the area under the curve 60% higher (85.2 *vs.* 53.5 μmol/L) and urinary output 100% greater (1.40 *vs.* 0.70 μmol/mg creatinine). In addition, the differences in bioavailability remained the same between the enteric-coated tablets and the nonenteric-coated capsules when they were both administered concurrently with the calcium carbonate capsules used in the Mayo Clinic study (12). If we take overall account of the high dose, the high bioavailability, and the long duration of the study, the cumulative dose of fluoride taken up by bone can be estimated to be more than 3 times as great as the total reached at the end of the French INSERM study (3). It is well known that bone fluoride content increases linearly with the duration of the treatment for an identical oral dose (13), and that a high cumulative dose of NaF can induce severe mineralization defect in bone tissue. Kleerekoper *et al.* (14) have recently shown that osteomalacia (defined as an osteoid volume higher than 5% and a mineralization lag time longer than 100 days) was found in 69% of 13 osteoporotic patients who had received 75 mg/day of NaF for a mean duration of 42 months. It is likely that the increased vertebral fracture rate noted during the third and fourth years of treatment in the Mayo Clinic trial could be due to toxic effects of fluoride on bone tissue and bone cells, with a significant miner-alization defect and also toxic effects on the osteoblast population, similar to those found in skeletal fluorosis (15). The publication of data on bone fluoride content and histomorphometric findings from the Mayo Clinic study will be of major interest. The mean serum fluoride and urinary fluoride levels reported in Riggs' paper (and expressed in μmol/liter) do not reflect the actual levels present in patients, because NaF administration was stopped 48 hours before the blood was drawn for serum fluoride and 24 hours before the 24-hour urine was collected (BL Riggs, personal communication).

If a mineralization defect is confirmed in the patients long term treated in the Mayo Clinic trial, this could explain the absence of a significant relationship between the increase in vertebral density and the changes in fracture rate reported by the authors (16), because of the presence of marked abnormalities in bone quality. In contrast, in a recent large study on 514 patients treated for a mean duration of 29 months with a dose of 29 mg elemental fluoride/day, Farley *et al.* (17) have shown that the lumbar fracture rate was inversely related to spinal bone density measured by quantitative computed tomography. Fluoride-treated patients exhibiting a sig-nificant increase in lumbar bone density had a 70% reduction in lumbar fracture rate compared to nonresponders. If we analyze the potential of fluoride therapy to restore trabecular bone mass in light of the "fracture threshold" concept, it is important to realize that a major increase in bone mass, even of 50% or 100%, will be unable to achieve a protective effect on further vertebral fractures if the initial trabecular bone volume is extremely low. In the Mayo Clinic study (4) where the mean lumbar bone mineral density (LBMD) was 0.77 g/cm^2 in the fluoride group, the 35% mean increase in LBMD only brought the mean value approximately to the level of the fracture threshold. This means that about 50% of patients after 4 years of treatment still had a LBMD lower than the "fracture threshold" value. It also means that any late intervention on bones where major rarefaction of trabeculae and near destruction of the trabecular network are already present is of little use in preventing further fractures. This should encourage earlier intervention in osteoporotic patients.

The reduction in vertebral fracture rate in osteoporotic patients treated long term with enteric-coated NaF tablets has recently been confirmed by two open studies by Franke and Hauch and Hodsman *et al.*, both presented during the 3rd International Symposium on Osteoporosis (Copenhagen; October 14–20, 1990). Franke and Hauch (18) have treated 52 osteoporotic patients for 2 to 5 years with 60 to 80 mg NaF/day. The fracture rate was 750 fractures/1,000 patient years in the first year and fell to 96 in the second year and to zero in the third and fourth years. Hodsman *et al.* (19) have treated 55 patients with NaF in daily doses of 20 to 60 mg. Vertebral fracture rate was 318/1,000 patient years in responders and 632/1,000 in nonresponders during the interval between 18 and 36 months ($p < 0.01$). The patients classified as responders had an average change of 7% to 8% over baseline vertebral bone mineral density. During the first 18 months of treatment the vertebral fracture rate was identical in nonresponders and responders (576 and 578/1,000, respectively).

SIDE EFFECTS

All open studies have shown that fluoride therapy may induce side effects, particularly gastrointestinal and osteoarticular, and both appear to be dose-related.

Gastrointestinal

Gastrointestinal side effects occur in 10% to 40% of patients. They commonly include nausea and vomiting and, very rarely, anemia due to blood loss. In the French INSERM study using a low dose of enteric-coated Osteofluor tablets (3), the relative risk of gastrointestinal disorders (non-NaF/NaF) was found to be 1.08 (non-significant) after adjustment for a history of digestive disorders. In the Mayo Clinic study using a high dose and nonenteric-coated capsules (4), the fluoride-treated women had gastric symptoms 2.9 times more frequently than the women given placebo. In contrast, in a recent study using a slow-release sodium fluoride tablet (25 mg twice daily) given as an intermittent treatment for 3 out of 5 months, less than 15% of patients had adverse gastrointestinal reactions (20).

Osteoarticular

From published reports, transient lower extremity pain is experienced by 10% to 50% of treated patients. In the French study, episodes of osteoarticular pain were frequent in both groups of patients followed for 2 years: 37% of fluoride-treated patients *versus* 30% of non-fluoride subjects (3). Pain in the ankle and foot were, however, noted significantly more often among fluoride-treated patients than in the non-fluoride group: 15% of patients in the NaF group compared with 5% in the non-NaF group had at least one episode of pain in the ankle and foot ($p < 0.01$). In the US study (4), lower extremity pain syndrome occurred in 37 patients receiving NaF and in five receiving placebo. About 10% of the episodes were bilateral. In a study comparing NaF (50 mg/day of Osteofluor) and monofluorophosphate (MFP, 200 mg/day), Delmas *et al.* (21) noted that the incidence of lower extremity pain related to stress microfractures was significantly higher with MFP than with NaF (34.5% *vs.* 15.4%, $p < 0.05$). The number of episodes per patient years of treatment was also greater in the MFP group (36.8% *vs.* 12.5%, $p < 0.01$). Patients who developed lower extremity pain had a greater increase in lumbar bone mineral density than those who did not. These differences have been shown to be related to a much better bio-availability of fluoride when given as MFP (100-mg effervescent tablet) than when given as a 25-mg enteric-coated tablet of NaF. In an open study using intermittent treatment with a slow-release fluoride preparation, Pak *et al.* found 14% of patients had rheumatic complaints (22).

Non-vertebral Fractures: Effects of Fluoride on Cortical Bone

Non-vertebral fractures—in particular hip fractures—have been found to be more frequent in patients treated with fluoride in some uncontrolled studies (23,24), whereas in other studies the incidence of these fractures has not been affected (3,25). They occurred with equal frequency in the two groups followed for 2 years in the INSERM French trial (3): 24 fractures were noted in the NaF group (including six hip fractures) and 22 in the non-NaF group (including four hip fractures). In the total population of 446 patients, 28 fractures were reported in each group, including seven hip fractures in the NaF group and eight in the non-NaF group. In the Mayo Clinic trial (4), the number of complete fractures was not significantly different between the two groups, with seven hip fractures (including one traumatic fracture) in the NaF-calcium group and three in the calcium group. In the Henry Ford Hospital trial (6), two hip fractures occurred in the calcium group and three in the NaF-calcium group. In the Mayo Clinic trial, the bone mineral density decreased by 1% per year in the shaft of the radius containing predominantly cortical bone (minus 4% in 4 years; $p < 0.02$). This confirms the results obtained by Hodsman and Drost (26) with 60 mg/day of NaF given for 29 months on average. They reported that cortical bone density in the forearm decreased by an alarming 7.7%/year. This was not the case in our first study using 50 mg/day of NaF for 2 years, where radial bone mineral content did not change (27). Schulz *et al.* (28) have recently evaluated the effect of fluoride therapy on cortical thickness in 52 osteoporotic patients by separately measuring cortical and trabecular densities in the first lumbar vertebra with quantitative computed tomography. They found an increase in trabecular bone density of 3.20

± 1.87 mg/ml (value ± SD) per month and a corresponding increase in cortical bone density of 3.17 ± 2.14 mg/ml per month. A paired *t* test analysis showed that the differences between the trabecular and cortical rates of increase were not significant. In addition, Strauss *et al.* (29), studying 28 patients with postmenopausal osteoporosis for an average of 2.2 years after the discontinuation of NaF therapy given for an average of 4.6 years at a mean dose of 44 ± 9 mg/day of NaF (enteric-coated), have shown that the non-vertebral fracture rate was not increased. While on NaF, this non-vertebral fracture rate was 154 fractures/1,000 patient years and was not significantly different after NaF was discontinued (129 fractures/1,000 patient years). In the meantime, they have shown that the increase in mineral mass, expressed as the calcium/bone index (CaBI), was largely maintained after NaF was discontinued.

In a recent study, Pouilles *et al.* (30) have analyzed the effects of a daily treatment with 50 mg NaF (enteric-coated Osteofluor 25), 1 g calcium, and 400 IU vitamin D_2 on both vertebral and femoral bone densities in 52 postmenopausal osteopenic women. They found a 5.5% increase in vertebral bone density at 24 months in the NaF group and a 1.8% decrease in the control group, while femoral neck and trochanteric bone mineral density declined by 2% to 3%, without any difference between the NaF and control groups.

CONCLUSION

Since 1987, the results of two large controlled trials made in the United States (4,6) have shown that high daily doses of sodium fluoride (75 mg) given in nonenteric-coated capsules, providing high bioavailability of fluoride, do not provide a valid benefit-to-risk ratio in 4 years of treatment of established vertebral osteoporosis. They had a limited efficacy and induced a large number of side effects, with histological evidence of a mineralization defect in two-thirds of the patients (14). This corresponds to a cumulative dose delivered to bone that is about 3 times greater than the one provided by a 50-mg daily dose given in enteric-coated tablets for 2 years. Bone fluoride content is known to increase linearly with the duration of treatment in osteoporosis or with the time of exposure in toxic skeletal fluorosis, and the incidence of osteoarticular side effects is clearly dose-dependent, as shown by the analysis of the recently published reports. In contrast, all these studies—including two recent British open studies (31,32)—show that low doses (50 mg) of sodium fluoride given in enteric-coated tablets, providing much lower bioavailability of fluoride than nonenteric-coated capsules, are beneficial when given for 2 or 3 years in osteoporotic patients and have an acceptable incidence of side effects. These low doses are capable of reducing the vertebral fracture rate without increasing cortical bone loss and the non-vertebral fracture incidence. This has still to be proven for fluoride preparations having a higher bioavailability and/or containing a higher amount of fluoride ion, such as monofluorophosphate preparations.

Until recently, the message concerning the benefit-to-risk ratio of fluoride therapy in vertebral osteoporosis has been rather confusing, because "fluoride" has been taken into consideration globally without taking into account the fact that quite different therapeutic strategies have used different fluoride salts, different doses, different preparations providing very different bioavailabilities of fluoride ion, and different durations of treatment. NaF given as enteric-coated tablets and used at a daily dose of 50 mg, or MFP given as effervescent tablet and used at a daily dose of 150 to 200 mg, meet the conditions of dosage and bioavailability that correspond to an efficient and safe therapeutic window.

Because most studies with those compounds have lasted 2 years, the recommended duration of the treatment could be provisionally limited to 2 years. They should be given in combination with calcium supplements, while taking into account the classical contraindications: renal failure, osteomalacia, and previous hip fracture. The treatment should be prescribed as soon as possible after the first vertebral crush fracture.

REFERENCES

1. Watts NB, Harris ST, Genant HK, *et al.* Intermittent cyclical etidronate treatment of postmenopausal osteoporosis. *N Engl J Med* 1990;323:73–9.
2. Consensus development conference: prophylaxis and treatment of osteoporosis. *BMJ* 1987;295: 914–5.
3. Mamelle N, Meunier PJ, Dusan R, *et al.* Risk-benefit ratio of sodium fluoride treatment in primary vertebral osteoporosis. *Lancet* 1988;ii:361–4.
4. Riggs BL, Hodgson SF, O'Fallon WH, *et al.* Effect of fluoride treatment on the fracture rate in postmenopausal women with osteoporosis. *N Engl J Med* 1990;322:802–9.
5. Murray TM, Singer FR, eds. Proceedings of the International Workshop on Fluoride and Bone. *J Bone Miner Res* 1990;5:suppl 1.
6. Kleerekoper M, Peterson E, Philips E, Nelson D, Tilley B, Parfitt AM. Continuous sodium fluoride therapy does not reduce vertebral fracture rate in postmenopausal osteoporosis. *J Bone Miner Res* 1989;4(suppl 1):abstract 376.
7. Mamelle N, Meunier PJ, Netter P. Fluoride and vertebral fractures. *Lancet* 1990;336:243.
8. Kanis JA. Effect of fluoride on postmenopausal osteoporosis. *N Engl J Med* 1990;323:416.
9. Mallette LE. Effect of fluoride on postmenopausal osteoporosis. *N Engl J Med* 1990;323:417.
10. Nagant de Deuxchaisnes C, Devogelaer JP, Stein F. Fluoride treatment and vertebral fractures. *Lancet* 1990;336:48.
11. Heaney RP, Baylink DJ, Johnston CC, *et al.* Fluoride therapy for the vertebral crush fracture. *Ann Intern Med* 1989;8:678–80.
12. Nagant de Deuxchaisnes C, Devogelaer JP, Stein F. Comparison of the bioavailability of the NaF capsules used in the NIH sponsored trials as compared to that of NaF enteric-coated tablets commercially available in Europe. *J Bone Miner Res* 1990;5(suppl 2):abstract 710.
13. Boivin G, Chapuy MC, Baud CA, Meunier PJ. Fluoride content in human iliac bone: results in controls, patients with fluoride and osteoporosis patients treated with fluoride. *J Bone Miner Res* 1988;3:497–501.
14. Kleerekoper M, Balena R, Foldes J, Shih MS, Rao D, Parfitt AM. Histomorphometric changes in iliac bone induced by sodium fluoride therapy depend on cumulative dose. *J Bone Miner Res* 1990;5(suppl 2):abstract 267.
15. Boivin G, Chavassieux P, Chapuy MC, Baud CA, Meunier PJ. Skeletal fluorosis: histomorphometric analysis of bone changes and bone fluoride content in 29 patients. *Bone* 1989;10:89–99.
16. Riggs BL, Hodgson SF, O'Fallon WH, *et al.* Effects of fluoride on postmenopausal osteoporosis. *N Engl J Med* 1990;323:416–7.
17. Farley SM, Wergedal JE, Farley JR, *et al.* Fluoride decreases spinal fracture rate; a study of over 500 patients. In: Christiansen C, Overgaard K, eds. *Osteoporosis 1990.* Copenhagen: Osteopress, 1991:1330–4.

18. Franke J, Hauch S. Fractures and stress-fractures during NaF therapy. In: Christiansen C, Overgaard K, eds. *Osteoporosis 1990*. Copenhagen: Osteopress, 1991:1479–83.
19. Hodsman AB, Drost DJ, Goldenberg J. Reduced vertebral fracture rate in osteoporotic patients responding to fluoride treatment with an increasing vertebral bone mineral density. In: Christiansen C, Overgaard K, eds. *Osteoporosis 1990*. Copenhagen: Osteopress, 1991:1484–5.
20. Pak CYC, Sakhee K, Zerwekh JE. Effect of intermittent therapy with a slow release fluoride preparation. *J Bone Miner Res* 1990;5(suppl 1):149–55.
21. Delmas PD, Dupuis J, Duboeuf F, Chapuy MC, Meunier PJ. Treatment of vertebral osteoporosis with disodium monofluorophosphate: comparison with sodium fluoride. *J Bone Miner Res* 1990;5(suppl 1):143–7.
22. Pak CYC, Sakhee K, Zerwekh JE, Parcel C, Peterson R, Johnson K. A safe and primary osteoporosis by intermittent application of slow-release sodium fluoride. *J Clin Endocrinol Metab* 1989;68:150–9.
23. Gutteridge DH, Price RI, Nicholson GC, *et al*. Fluoride in osteoporotic vertebral fracture: trabecular increase, vertebral protection, femoral fracture. In: Christiansen C, *et al*. eds. *Osteoporosis 1984*. Copenhagen: Osteopress 1, 1984:705–7.
24. Hedlund LR, Gallagher JC. Increased incidence of hip fracture in osteoporotic women treated with sodium fluoride. *J Bone Miner Res* 1989;4:223–5.
25. Riggs BL, Baylink DJ, Kleerekoper M, Lane JM, Melton III LJ, Meunier PJ. Incidence of hip fractures in osteoporotic women treated with sodium fluoride. *J Bone Miner Res* 1987;2:123–6.
26. Hodsman AB, Drost DJ. The response of vertebral bone mineral density during treatment of osteoporosis with sodium fluoride. *J Clin Endocrinol Metab* 1989;69:932–8.
27. Briancon D, Meunier PJ. Treatment of osteoporosis with fluoride, calcium and vitamin D. *Orthop Clin North Am* 1981;12:629–48.
28. Schulz EE, Frykman G, Baylink DJ. Fluoride therapy increases bone density of cortical as well as trabecular bone of the vertebral body in patients with osteoporosis. In: Christiansen C, Overgaard K, eds. *Osteoporosis 1990*. Copenhagen: Osteopress, 1991:1386–8.
29. Strauss A, Bayley TA, Harrison JE, *et al*. Follow-up of osteoporotic patients after discontinuation of fluoride treatment. In: Christiansen C, Overgaard K, eds. *Osteoporosis 1990*. Copenhagen: Osteopress, 1991:1369–71.
30. Pouilles JM, Trémollières F, Causse E, Louvet JP, Ribot C. Fluoride therapy in postmenopausal osteopenic women: effect on vertebral and femoral bone density and prediction of bone response. *Osteoporosis Int* 1991;1:103–9.
31. Buckle RM. Three year study of sodium fluoride treatment on vertebral fracture incidence in osteoporosis. *J Bone Miner Res* 1989;4(suppl 1):abstract 275.
32. Wassif W, Pitt P, Li F, *et al*. Enteric-coated sodium fluoride for osteoporosis. Bone and Tooth Society. Spring meeting, 15th April 1991, abstract P14.

DISCUSSION

This chapter was part of the Round-Table Conference on prevention of osteoporosis. Please refer to the round-table discussion, page 187.

Nutrition of the Elderly, edited by H. Munro, and
G. Schlierf, Nestlé Nutrition Workshop Series, Vol. 29,
Nestec Ltd., Vevey/Raven Press, Ltd., New York © 1992.

Round-Table Discussion on Prevention of Osteoporosis

Dr. Hodkinson: I should like to ask Dr. Bonjour whether, in his second study where he was comparing protein versus no protein supplements, the supplements were of equal energy value.

Dr. Bonjour: There was a difference of 10% in the total energy consumed between the two groups.

Dr. Hodkinson: In your first study, your supplement, which was highly successful, provided around 15% to 20% additional energy, so if there was an energy imbalance of 10% in your second study, it could be significant.

Dr. Rush: I am concerned about the subjectivity of the end-points. Although the patients obviously could not be blinded to their treatment, some observers could have been. Did you use any other end-points apart from length of hospital stay, which seems to me to be very insecure since it could be affected by knowledge of treatment on the part of both the patients and the care-givers?

Dr. Bonjour: What suggestions do you have, accepting that double blinding is impossible?

Dr. Rush: There are various intermediate strategies. For example, the study could be single blinded to a set of observers who were asked to do an objective assessment of nutritional status or functional status, or whatever indices you accept as being relevant to the effect of the protein supplement. The length of hospital stay is not an end-point I am comfortable with, unsupported by other end-points.

Dr. Bonjour: Your point is well taken. We are not saying that what we have presented here is the end of the story. Other studies need to be done to confirm what we have found, using different outcome variables as you propose. Another thing we have not touched on is the mechanism; I think we need to measure possible mediators such as insulin-like growth factor (IGF) in these patients.

Dr. Guesry: It is said that peak bone mass is acquired between the 16th and 21st years of life. This rather implies that after 20 years of age nothing much can be done to improve the situation and delay the occurrence of hip fracture. What is your view on this? Should teenagers be advised to take more vitamin D and bone minerals? They don't worry much about what is likely to happen 50 years later!

Dr. Bonjour: I'm not sure that we really know at what time of life we can obtain most benefit from giving additional nutrients such as calcium. We need longitudinal data showing that enrichment of the diet with calcium and perhaps energy during the rapid phase of bone mass accumulation is effective in increasing bone mass. Studies in monozygotic twins have shown an effect of calcium supplementation but it is rather small and only certain areas of the skeleton appear to be significantly affected. Between the ages of 20 and 45, the period when bone mass seems to be more or less stable no study has so far demonstrated a major change in bone mass by supplementation or by exercise. As far as the elderly are concerned, I should like to have Dr. Meunier's comments because he has interesting data on supplementing elderly people with calcium and vitamin D.

Dr. Meunier: In parallel with the exponential increase in incidence of femoral fractures after the age of 80, there is continuing bone loss. We have shown recently in a cross-sectional and prospective study that the bone loss at the upper end of the femur is of the order of 2% to 3% per year until death and is associated with very high parathyroid hormone (PTH) values. When ambulatory elderly people with high levels of PTH are treated with supplements of calcium and vitamin D_2 or D_3, the PTH values fall by about 45% in 18 months and there is a cessation of bone loss from the upper femur. So it is never too late—we can still protect bone after the age of 80 with vitamin D and calcium supplements.

Dr. Berry: Since bone density depends on both calcium and bone matrix, which is protein collagen, is there any evidence that a low protein intake, in the presence of an adequate calcium intake, can lead to osteoporosis?

Dr. Bonjour: From what I know about the relationship between protein and osteoporosis in several human studies, I think it is very difficult to isolate protein from other nutrients in terms of individual responsibility for low bone mass.

Dr. Lindsay: I should like to comment on the hip fracture issue. Bone mass is a risk factor for hip fracture but it does not diagnose hip fracture, and the concept of bone mass separating fracture from nonfracture cases is of no great importance. When examining data in which people with hip fractures have been compared with age-matched controls, it is apparent that all old people have a low bone mass, so all are at risk of fracture. In cross-sectional data you are comparing those who have had a chance occurrence with those who are waiting for that chance occurrence to happen. Everyone who lives long enough, be they male or female, black or white, will become osteoporotic and will be at risk of fracture. At the same time, because they are getting older they will have an increased risk of falling and fallers are the ones most likely to get fractures.

Dr. Steen: I have a question for all the participants about the relative importance of different risk factors for osteoporosis. Judging from our longitudinal studies, we are of the firm opinion that there are two main risk factors and these are physical inactivity and smoking. Compared to these, the other known risks (calcium, estrogen, and so on) are relatively unimportant. Smoking has not been focused on as much as it should have been in this conference. When, in our analysis, we keep physical activity, alcohol intake, and body weight constant, we have a 30% difference between smokers and non-smokers in bone mineral content at age 70 years. Smoking is an important risk factor for osteoporosis.

Dr. Lindsay: I don't think anyone would disagree that smoking is a risk factor. However, if we look at this from the point of view of behavior modification, it is evident that it is very difficult to get people to give up smoking, even when they are threatened with much more serious risks than osteoporosis.

One of the concerns I have about bone mass as an outcome variable for interventions such as physical activity, nutrition, and so on, is that the methodology of bone mass measurement is very dependent on body composition. Thus, the changes one sees, if not adequately corrected for differences in body composition, will result in apparent differences that are perhaps much greater than the real differences.

Dr. Guesry: At a recent symposium in Lausanne on the prevention of osteoporosis, a group from Zurich reported on risk factors. Cigarette smoking appeared to play only a small role. Do you have any theory on the possible mode of action?

Dr. Steen: No, I don't. It is of course possible that there may be confounding factors and that smokers have other characteristics that put them at risk for osteoporosis. However, when we try to hold the other known factors constant in the analysis, there are still very large differences in bone mineral content between smokers and non-smokers at age 70 years.

Dr. Edwardson: I wonder what proportion of women in the age range of 70 to 75 years are smokers. I thought it was relatively small.

Dr. Steen: Although the proportion of smokers among women is definitely lower than among men, it is showing a dangerously increasing trend, in my country at least. Young women smoke very much more now than they did a couple of decades ago.

Dr. Lindsay: For the most part, of course, cigarette smokers don't live long enough to get hip fractures. However, it is worth recalling that smoking is associated with changes in estrogen metabolism resulting in a reduction in endogenous estrogen supply, perhaps making the need for exogenous estrogen greater.

Dr. Edwardson: Repeated studies in Newcastle and elsewhere in the United Kingdom have shown that 25% of hip fracture patients are severely demented and a further 50% show significant cognitive impairment. This is not simply a post-traumatic confusional state because repeat studies 6 months later show virtually the same cognitive test scores. In case there might be some underlying relationship between negative calcium balance and cognitive impairment, we have looked at bone mass in severely demented hip fracture patients in comparison with hip fracture patients of the same age with normal cerebral function and there is no difference at all. This suggests that the crucial risk factor is the predisposition toward falling related to cerebral impairment.

Dr. Lindsay: I hope I didn't give the impression that the answer to hip fracture is necessarily a pharmacologic intervention targeting the skeleton. That is one factor in the hip fracture equation. There is no doubt that falling is also an important factor, particularly in the nursing home population. However, falling is not a factor in vertebral crush fracture risk, and this type of fracture occurs in people going about normal daily activities. I think that the prevention of bone loss is likely to be important in reducing the incidence of all fractures.

Dr. Rush: It seems fairly clear that estrogen therapy is now being used widely and for prolonged periods, but what is known of the ultimate cost-effectiveness of estrogen in relation to osteoporosis and also in relation to other diseases such as cardiovascular diseases and cancer of the breast? What is the balance of risks associated with long-term estrogen therapy?

Dr. Lindsay: The epidemiological data are consistent in showing that the use of estrogens by themselves is associated with a reduction in the relative risk of cardiovascular disease in postmenopausal women. This may in part be related to changes in lipoprotein metabolism. The reduction in risk of death from cardiovascular disease, which is the most common cause of death in postmenopausal women in the United States, is of the order of 50% with estrogen therapy. However, it must also be said that the use of estrogen alone increases the relative risk of developing endometrial cancer by two- to eightfold. Survival from endometrial cancer is almost 100%, and the survival in estrogen-treated women is even greater than in women who have not received estrogens, for reasons I don't completely understand.

The issue of breast cancer is much more complicated and potentially problematic. My conclusions from the currently available data are that estrogens increase the risk of breast cancer by between 10% and 30% when treatment has been given for prolonged periods, that is, 10 years or more. There are data to show that the increased risk ceases to be present when estrogens are discontinued, which leaves me rather concerned about the mechanism. The implications of these data are that the risk of developing breast cancer in the average postmenopausal woman of 50, which is normally about 1:9, will increase to 1:8. Since breast cancer is so common, this represents a fairly important increase in the potential total numbers of malignancies. However, I am unaware of any studies that have shown higher mortality from breast cancer in estrogen-treated postmenopausal women, and in fact several show decreased mortality. The reason that women *discontinue* estrogen replacement therapy in the United States has little to do with cancer. It is because cyclical menstrual bleeding is socially unacceptable after the age of 50. Until we find a mechanism for prescribing estrogen, with or without progestin, that does not produce endometrial bleeding, this will continue to be a problem.

Dr. Rush: I think the apparent disparity between incidence and survival in the breast cancer data is not something I should be at all confident in. It has been shown clearly that women who receive estrogens are from a different social class background and are exposed to a different level of medical care.

Dr. Lindsay: There is no doubt that part of the survival difference is related to detection by physicians; that is, women on estrogen are more likely to have a malignancy diagnosed at an early stage because it is looked for.

Dr. Glick: I am not clear about whether there is information on the net effect of exercise on bone strength.

Dr. Meredith: The final message is that exercise, if it is frequent enough and vigorous enough, will affect bone density at any age, just as immobilization will affect it in the other direction at any age. In young military conscripts exposed to heavy physical training schedules, the increase in bone density is of the order of 11% over a period of weeks, although a number of recruits suffer fractures. It appears that we need to balance the amount of exercise taken such that it is sufficient to increase bone density without causing fractures.

Dr. Glick: Is the regular exercise involved in normal day-to-day activities meaningful in maintaining bone structure?

Dr. Meredith: Your bone mass is appropriate for a certain level of exercise. If you decrease your level of exercise bone mass will also decrease, but no further than a certain set point. If you abruptly increase or decrease your habitual exercise the bone mass set point will change.

Dr. Chen: What about medications as risk factors for osteoporosis? I am concerned particularly about diuretics, which may deplete calcium.

Dr. Lindsay: Medications are important causes of secondary osteoporosis, not only diuretics but also overtreatment with thyroid hormone (even when given as replacement therapy), and of course glucocorticoids. One problem related to calcium deficiency is that we don't really know how to define it since there is no test for it.

Dr. Guesry: Don't you think that secondary (presumably) hyperparathyroidism is a good indicator of calcium deficiency?

Dr. Lindsay: I don't think it is sensitive enough. Although there is an adaptive mechanism to increase calcium absorption in the face of calcium deficiency, involving increased PTH and stimulation of $1,25(OH)_2D$, this varies considerably from person to person, and PTH may not go outside the normal range in some people with calcium deficiency.

Dr. Chen: The RDA for calcium was revised in 1989. According to the revised values, the RDA for a woman of 50 is 800 mg. Is this an adequate amount for a woman in this age group?

Dr. Bonjour: I think 800 mg is probably enough but there are many studies showing that in the 5 years after menopause even if you increase the calcium intake to 1,200 or 1,300 mg per day you cannot stop the bone loss, so maybe we should be giving even more.

Dr. Guesry: Is there any information about the effect of fluoridation of water supplies on bone mineralization?

Dr. Meunier: A study was reported in the *Lancet* by Simonen and Laitinen (1) in which they investigated the effect of water supplemented to a level of 1 mg fluoride ion per liter. There was a lower incidence of femoral fracture in the group receiving this small dose.

Dr. Guesry: This is quite encouraging because this level of fluoridation is free of side effects.

Dr. Meunier: Some mineral waters available in France are rich in fluoride. We have investigated 23 heavy drinkers of one particular variety of mineral water containing 8.5 mg fluoride ion per liter, which is a lot. We found a significant increase in lumbar bone mineral density in these people without any symptoms of fluorosis.

REFERENCE

1. Simonen O, Laitinen O. Does fluoridation of drinking water prevent bone fragility and osteoporosis. *Lancet* 1985;ii:432–4.

Nutrition of the Elderly, edited by H. Munro, and
G. Schlierf, Nestlé Nutrition Workshop Series, Vol. 29,
Nestec Ltd., Vevey/Raven Press, Ltd., New York © 1992.

Alzheimer's Disease and Brain Mineral Metabolism

James A. Edwardson

Medical Research Council Neurochemical Pathology Unit, Newcastle General Hospital, Newcastle upon Tyne NE4 6BE, England, UK

Dementia constitutes one of the greatest medical and social problems facing the aging populations of developed countries. Alzheimer's disease is the main cause of dementia in the elderly, and the cognitive decline that characterizes this disorder clinically is accompanied by the development of hallmark neuropathological changes, including loss of neurons and synapses and the development of senile plaques and neurofibrillary tangles. Plaques consist of extracellular deposits of an abnormal protein fragment, the β-amyloid peptide, which aggregates in fibrils in a "star-burst" array to form the core of mature plaques. This plaque core is surrounded by neuritic processes and glial cells and there is loss of synapses in the adjacent neuropil (1).

Neurofibrillary tangles are lesions in which paired helical filaments (PHFs) are deposited intracellularly. A major component of PHFs is an abnormally phosphorylated form of the microtubule-associated protein, tau, indicating a derangement of cytoskeletal function in affected neurons (2).

THE ETIOPATHOGENESIS OF ALZHEIMER'S DISEASE

It seems likely that Alzheimer's disease has a complex etiology and that, in common with many other disorders, both genetic and environmental factors may be important. Genetic linkage studies have provided evidence of heterogeneity and some presenile familial forms show linkage to chromosome 21, while others do not (3). A rare familial form involves a base substitution in the gene encoding the β-amyloid precursor protein (APP) located on chromosome 21 (4). However, the majority of late onset cases of Alzheimer's disease appear to be sporadic and it seems likely that environmental factors are important in this condition.

Environmental agents, including nutritional factors, could in theory contribute to the development of Alzheimer's disease in two main ways. According to the "threshold model" of neurodegenerative disorders (5), there is an age-related general attrition of neuronal systems with loss of functional capacity, due to the combined effects of genetic and environmental factors. Superimposed on this decline, a more

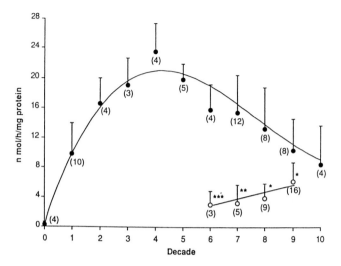

FIG. 1. Choline acetyltransferase in the hippocampus of intellectually normal individuals (•) and Alzheimer cases (o). This pattern is consistent with the "threshold model" for neurodegenerative disorders, the disease in older patients being expressed against a background of increased general involutional change, so that clinical symptoms may occur with a correspondingly smaller deficit in cholinergic function. The zero position on the decade scale represents preterm cases before cholinergic innervation is established ($^*p < 0.05$, $^{**}p < 0.02$, $^{***}p < 0.001$).

specific disease process causes accelerated neuronal cell death or dysfunction until the threshold for adaptive compensation is exceeded and clinical symptoms develop. This is illustrated in Fig. 1, which shows age-related changes in the hippocampal content of choline acetyltransferase (ChAT), the enzyme responsible for acetylcholine synthesis, in intellectually normal individuals. Memory loss, a core clinical symptom of Alzheimer's disease, correlates well with the severe decline in ChAT and other markers of cholinergic function in the hippocampus and neocortex (6). Figure 1 also shows levels of ChAT in patients with Alzheimer's disease and it is evident that the later the onset of the disorder, the less the levels of ChAT are reduced. This pattern is consistent with the threshold model, the disease in older subjects being expressed against a greater burden of general involutional change, resulting in clinical symptoms with a correspondingly smaller deficit in cholinergic function. A growing body of evidence suggests that alterations in brain mineral homeostasis may play a role in the development of Alzheimer's disease and a key issue is whether these changes account for part of the general age-related attrition of brain function or whether they contribute more specifically to the etiopathogenesis of the disorder.

THE ROLE OF ALUMINUM

Involvement of aluminum in the etiopathogenesis of Alzheimer's disease is suggested by several lines of evidence. Aluminum is associated with both of the characteristic neuropathological lesions, the plaques and tangles. The Al content of tangle-bearing neurons is increased compared to that of adjacent non-tangled neurons (7). Studies in susceptible animal species have shown that Al induces the abnormal phosphorylation of neurofilament proteins (8), an aberration similar to that which occurs in the hyperphosphorylated form of tau associated with PHFs in Alzheimer's disease (2). Aluminum in the form of amorphous aluminosilicate is present at the center of the β-amyloid core in mature senile plaques (9,10) and such deposits have not been found associated with other neuropathological lesions or systemic amyloid deposits (11). Although these changes have not been consistently found by some other groups, we have argued that this is probably due to methodological problems and have confirmed the presence of Al in plaque cores using a variety of techniques including both energy and wavelength dispersive scanning electron microprobe x-ray analysis, scanning proton microprobe x-ray microanalysis, and imaging secondary ion mass spectrometry (SIMS).

Aluminum in the circulation is mainly, if not completely, bound to the iron-transporting protein transferrin and entry to the brain appears to be largely via this route (12,13). Accumulation of Al occurs in regions of the brain that contain high densities of transferrin receptors, notably in regions such as cortex, hippocampus, and amygdala, which are selectively vulnerable in Alzheimer's disease.

Immunocytochemical staining for the transferrin receptor reveals high densities on pyramidal cells and other projection neurons that have the greatest requirement for iron in the synthesis of respiratory chain enzymes. Studies using imaging SIMS have shown high focal concentrations of Al with a laminar distribution corresponding to that of pyramidal neurons in the brains of patients with chronic renal failure (13). Such patients are exposed to high plasma levels of Al as a consequence of impaired renal excretion and chronic treatment with Al-containing phosphate binders to prevent hyperphosphatemia. Figure 2 illustrates the finding that cortical pyramidal neurons in dialysis patients show increased staining for the β-APP and also that approximately 30% of these patients exhibit precocious deposition of β-amyloid in the form of immature plaques (14). Although APP may be a "cell stress" protein, such changes have not been found in patients with hepatic encephalopathy, and β-amyloid deposition may thus be a direct response to the accumulation of toxic levels of Al in these cells.

Aluminum causes dialysis encephalopathy (15) and although the neuropathological changes in this condition do not resemble those in Alzheimer's disease, this probably reflects the severity and relatively acute form of exposure. The deposition of β-amyloid during senile plaque formation appears to occur over years and probably even decades (16), a time course consistent with the slow accumulation of aluminum in vulnerable neuronal populations that could lead to pathological changes including the increased expression or abnormal processing of APP. We have shown that the incidence of presenile Alzheimer's disease appears to be increased in areas where there are high levels of aluminum in water supplies (17) and similar findings have been reported from three other studies (18–20). This relationship is surprising in view of the relatively small proportion of dietary Al contributed by water, compared

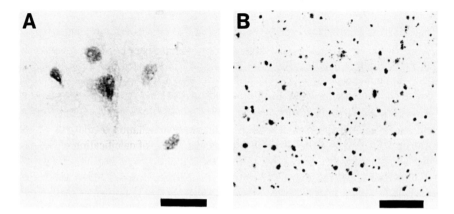

FIG. 2. Immunostaining for the β-APP associated with pyramidal cells in the cortex of a chronic renal dialysis patient (**A**) and the presence of immunostained immature plaques (**B**) in the cerebral cortex of the same patient. Increased staining for APP occurs in the vast majority of such patients exposed to aluminum, whereas plaque formation is evident only in about 30% of cases. Scale bar in A represents 20 μm and in B 500 μm.

with the much larger amounts from other sources including food additives, medicines, and substances such as tea, which are naturally rich in aluminum (21). One possible explanation is that the soluble forms of Al that result from water treatment may represent a particularly bioavailable source. However, Birchall has pointed out an alternative explanation that focuses on the important role of silicon in relation to aluminum toxicity.

THE ROLE OF SILICON IN ALUMINUM TOXICITY

Unlike aluminum, silicon appears to be an essential trace element and Birchall and Chappell have proposed that its main role in the body may be to limit the bioavailability of aluminum (22). They have also suggested that the epidemiological findings referred to above may be explained by the broad inverse relationship that exists between the content of Al and Si in water supplies and the ability of silicic acid, $Si(OH)_4$, the dissolved form of Si, to complex with Al^{3+} from other dietary sources and thus reduce the general bioavailability of aluminum (23). Silicon is present in serum as silicic acid and it is also present in cerebrospinal fluid (24). The solubility of $Si(OH)_4$ decreases markedly in the presence of Al, and aluminosilicate complexes can form at extracellular pH (22). Thus, high focal concentrations of Al released on neuronal cell death may complex with $Si(OH)_4$ in the extracellular fluid to form a focal deposit of aluminosilicate that could act as a nidus for plaque core formation. A significant increase in the cerebrospinal fluid content of Si in senile but not presenile Alzheimer's disease has been reported, and this correlated with the severity of functional impairment (24). This increase may reflect the accumulation of aluminum and development of core-containing senile plaques in which aluminosilicate deposits are present (9,10).

CALCIUM HOMEOSTASIS IN DEMENTIA

Altered cellular calcium homeostasis has been reported in Alzheimer's disease and could potentially contribute to neurodegenerative changes through effects such as those on cytoskeletal turnover and excitatory amino acid–mediated neurotoxicity. It has been proposed that the parkinsonism–dementia–ALS complex of Guam represents a form of secondary hyperparathyroidism due to chronic deficiency of calcium and magnesium, which results in increased accumulation of toxic metal ions in the nervous system (25). The prevalence and severity of calcification of the basal ganglia are greater in Down syndrome and in patients under 75 years of age with Alzheimer's disease, in comparison with age-matched controls. Cellular calcium content increases with age and is significantly elevated in the cortex of neuropathologically confirmed cases of Alzheimer's disease (26). There is evidence that changes in cellular calcium homeostasis may be present in peripheral tissue in Alzheimer's disease and reduced calcium uptake *in vitro* by skin fibroblasts and mitogen-stimulated lymphocytes has been reported. Using ^{45}Ca, we have recently shown that there is a marked decrease in the gastrointestinal absorption of calcium in Alzheimer patients and that this occurs in the presence of normal plasma concentrations of parathormone and vitamin D metabolites (27). However, similar changes were also found in patients with multi-infarct dementia, suggesting that this impairment is a non-specific derangement (Table 1). Furthermore, in an epidemiological study to determine whether the negative calcium balance of age-related osteoporosis predisposed to senile dementia, we have measured bone mass and cognitive function in elderly hip fracture patients (28). No correlation was evident between mental test score and bone mass in the proximal femur measured in 347 patients (Fig. 3). The results are consistent with the view that dementia is associated with an increased

TABLE 1. *Gastrointestinal absorption of calcium in dementia*

Group	Alzheimer's disease	Multi-infarct dementia	Controls
No.	26	11	24
Age	76 ± 7	76 ± 9	74 ± 5
Mental test score	9***	11***	26
Serum Ca (mmol/liter)	2.43 ± 0.13	2.35 ± 0.08	2.45 ± 0.1
Serum PTH (ng/ml)	0.8 ± 0.5	—	0.8 ± 0.3
1,25(OH)$_2$ vitamin D (pg/ml)	22 ± 12	—	20 ± 8
^{45}Ca absorption	0.29 ± 0.17**	0.38 ± 0.24*	0.6 ± 0.30

Absorption of radioactive calcium in Alzheimer's disease, multi-infarct dementia, and age-matched control subjects, measured using a method that takes weight into account and correlates well with dual isotope and metabolic balance studies (24). Reduced absorption of ^{45}Ca in Alzheimer's disease occurs in the presence of normal levels of parathormone and vitamin D metabolites. Means ± SD. * $p < 0.05$; ** $p < 0.01$; *** $p < 0.001$.

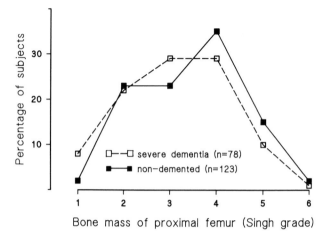

FIG. 3. Relationship between bone mass and cognitive function in the elderly: Bone mass of the proximal femur in 78 hip fracture patients with severe dementia and 123 intellectually normal fracture patients, showing similar pattern of distribution. The Singh grade is a measure of femoral neck trabecular pattern from grade 6, where all major trabeculae are present, to grade 1 in which only the primary compressive group is visible. A further 146 patients with mild to moderate dementia showed a similar pattern of distribution.

risk of falling rather than with any complex etiopathological hypothesis linking negative calcium balance, as evidenced by osteoporosis, with dementia in the elderly. These findings do not, of course, exclude the possibility that derangements of neuronal calcium homeostasis could have an important role in the development of degenerative changes associated with dementia.

IMPLICATIONS FOR NUTRITIONAL RESEARCH

Understanding the changes in brain mineral homeostasis that occur during brain aging and in dementing disorders is a major challenge for future research. This brief chapter has focused on the possible neurotoxic actions of aluminum accumulation in the nervous system, the poorly understood role of silicon in relation to aluminum toxicity, and age-related changes in calcium homeostasis. Alterations in the neuronal homeostasis of other elements such as iron, manganese, and zinc may be of equal importance and are also poorly understood. The potential of iron to promote hydroxyl ion free-radical formation and cell damage by lipid peroxidation in disorders such as Alzheimer's disease and Parkinson's disease is an important area for research. It is of interest that the first genetic mutation to be described for familial Alzheimer's disease (4) may involve disruption of a regulatory stem-loop structure in the messenger RNA for the β-APP (29). This stem-loop contains the consensus nucleotide sequence found in the iron-responsive elements in the genes that encode for ferritin and the transferrin receptor and, by analogy, may be a translational regulatory site that controls production of APP. If the synthesis of this key protein in Alzheimer-type pathology is regulated in some way by intracellular iron homeostasis, such a mechanism could provide a unifying hypothesis for the role of genetic and environmental factors in the etiopathogenesis of this disorder.

The evidence suggesting that aluminum may contribute to age-related neurodegenerative changes raises obvious questions for investigation. Whereas some dietary constituents, such as citrate, markedly enhance the gastrointestinal absorption of aluminum, others, such as phosphate, fluoride, polyphenolic organic groups, and silicic acid, may interact with Al to reduce absorption. It remains to be determined whether intervention through chelation therapy or the increased intake of $Si(OH)_4$, for example, will significantly decrease Al absorption and slow the progression of Alzheimer's disease. There may be age-related changes in the uptake, tissue distribution, and excretion of Al, and genetic or other constitutional factors that confer susceptibility in some individuals. A pilot study from this laboratory has indicated that Alzheimer patients below the age of 75 years show increased absorption of Al following an oral challenge with aluminum citrate compared with age-matched controls, whereas other work has suggested that the binding of [67]Ga (and by implication Al) to plasma transferrin may be altered in Alzheimer's disease and Down syndrome (30). The apparent lack of a correlation between bone mass and dementia (28) suggests that there is no direct relationship between the negative calcium balance of old age and the processes that underlie dementia, but cognitive studies in large cohorts of subjects treated to prevent osteoporosis may shed further light on this problem. The possibility that age-related increases in free-radical–mediated damage or APP gene expression may result from alterations in neuronal iron homeostasis is another key issue, since such mechanisms could, ultimately, afford the possibility of control via pharmacological and nutritional strategies.

REFERENCES

1. Masliah E, Terry RD, Mallory M, Alford M, Hansen LA. Diffuse plaques do not accentuate synapse loss in Alzheimer's disease. *Am J Pathol* 1990;137:1293–7.
2. Lee VM-Y, Balin BJ, Otvos L, Trojanowski JQ. A68: a major sub-unit of paired helical filaments and derivatized forms of normal tau. *Science* 1991;251:675–8.
3. St George-Hyslop PH, Haines JL, Farrer LA, *et al*. Genetic linkage studies suggest that Alzheimer's disease is not a single homogeneous disorder. *Nature* 1990;347:194–7.
4. Goate A, Chartier-Harlin M-C, Mullan M, *et al*. Segregation of a missense mutation in the amyloid precursor gene with familial Alzheimer's disease. *Nature* 1991;349:704–6.
5. McGeer PL, McGeer EG, Suzuki J, Nagai T. Aging, Alzheimer's disease and the cholinergic system of the basal forebrain. *Neurology* 1984;34:741–5.
6. Perry EK. The cholinergic hypothesis: ten years on. *Br Med Bull* 1986;42:63–9.
7. Perl DP, Brody AR. Alzheimer's disease: x-ray spectrometric evidence of aluminum accumulation in neurofibrillary tangle-bearing neurons. *Science* 1980;208:297–9.
8. Troncoso JC, Sternberger NH, Sternberger LA, Hoffman PN, Price DL. Immunocytochemical studies of neurofilament antigens in the neurofibrillary pathology induced by aluminum. *Brain Res* 1986;364:295–300.
9. Candy JM, Oakley AE, Klinowski J, *et al*. Aluminosilicates and senile plaque formation in Alzheimer's disease. *Lancet* 1986;i:354–7.
10. Edwardson JA, Klinowski J, Oakley AE, Perry RH, Candy JM. Aluminosilicates and the aging brain:

implications for the pathogenesis of Alzheimer's disease. In: *Silicon biochemistry*. Ciba Foundation Symposium 121. Chichester: John Wiley, 1986:160–79.

11. Candy JM, Oakley AE, Gauvreau D, *et al*. Association of aluminum and silicon with neuropathological changes in the ageing brain. *Interdisciplinary Topics Gerontol* 1988;25:140–55.

12. Pullen RGL, Candy JM, Morris CM, Taylor GA, Keith AB, Edwardson JA. Gallium-67 as a potential marker for aluminum transport in rat brain: implications for Alzheimer's disease. *J Neurochem* 1990;55:251–9.

13. Morris CM, Candy JM, Oakley AE, *et al*. Comparison of regional distribution of transferrin receptors and aluminum in the forebrain of chronic renal dialysis patients. *J Neurol Sci* 1989;94:295–306.

14. Edwardson JA, Candy JM. Aluminum and the pathogenesis of senile plaques: studies in Alzheimer's disease and chronic renal failure. *Environ Geochem Health* 1990;12:94–6.

15. Alfrey AC, LeGendre GR, Kaehny WD. The dialysis encephalopathy syndrome. Possible aluminum intoxication. *N Engl J Med* 1976;294:184–8.

16. Muller-Hill B, Beyreuther K. Molecular biology of Alzheimer's disease. *Annu Rev Biochem* 1989;58:287–307.

17. Martyn CN, Barker DJP, Osmond C, Harris EC, Edwardson JA, Lacey RF. Geographical relation between Alzheimer's disease and aluminum in drinking water. *Lancet* 1989;i:354–7.

18. Flaten TP. Geographical associations between aluminum in drinking water and death rates with dementia (including Alzheimer's disease), Parkinson's disease and amyotrophic lateral sclerosis in Norway. *Environ Geochem Health* 1990;12:152–68.

19. Michel P, Commenges D, Dartigues JF et al. Study of the relationship between aluminum concentration in drinking water and risk of Alzheimer's disease. In: Iqbal K, McLachlan DRC, Winblad B, et al. eds. *Alzheimer's disease: Basic mechanisms, diagnosis and therapeutic strategies*. Chichester: Wiley, 1991;387–91.

20. Neri LC, Hewitt D. Aluminum, Alzheimer's disease and drinking water. *Lancet* 1991;338–90.

21. Epstein SG. Human exposure to aluminum. *Environ Geochem Health* 1990;12:65–70.

22. Birchall JD, Chappell JS. The chemistry of aluminum in relation to Alzheimer's disease. *Clin Chem* 1988;34:265–7.

23. Birchall JD, Chappell JS. Aluminum, water chemistry and Alzheimer's disease. *Lancet* 1989;i:953.

24. Hershey LA, Hershey CO, Varnes HW. CSF silicon in dementia. *Neurology* 1984;34:1197–201.

25. Garruto RM, Yase Y. Neurodegenerative disorders of the Western Pacific: the search for mechanisms of pathogenesis. *Trends Neurosci* 1986;9:368–74.

26. Corrigan FM, Finlayson JD, Stevenson G, Ashcroft GW, Ward NI. Aluminum, zinc and other elements in senile dementia of Alzheimer type. *Trace Element Med* 1987;4:117–9.

27. Ferrier IN, Leake A, Taylor GA, McKeith IG, Fairbairn AF, Robinson CJ, Francis RM, Edwardson JA. Reduced gastrointestinal absorption of calcium in dementia. *Age Ageing* 1990;19:368–75.

28. Wood DJ, Cooper C, Stevens J, Edwardson JA. Bone mass and dementia in hip fracture patients from areas with different aluminum concentrations in water supplies. *Age Ageing* 1988;17:415–9.

29. Tanzi RE, Hyman BT. Alzheimer's mutation. *Nature* 1991;350:564.

30. Farrar G, Altmann P, Welch S, *et al*. Defective gallium-transferrin binding in Alzheimer's disease and Down syndrome: possible mechanism for accumulation of aluminum in brain. *Lancet* 1990;335:747–50.

DISCUSSION

Dr. Schiffman: One of the major theories about the entry of aluminum into the brain is that it occurs via the nasal mucosa. What is your view on this?

Dr. Edwardson: I would disagree about this being a major hypothesis for the entry of aluminum into the brain. As far as I am aware, this is a minority view. The experimental studies that have shown translocation of aluminum in various forms from the nasal epithelium into the brain have been experimental situations in which vast quantities of aluminum have been applied directly to the nasal epithelium. We have looked at the uptake of aluminum in the brains of renal dialysis patients using imaging secondary iron mass spectrometry and it is quite clear that one can see increased focal accumulation of aluminum in many areas, including the olfactory system. This suggests that the primary route of access of aluminum, even in olfactory structures, is probably via transferrin-mediated transport from the circulation rather than by direct inhalation and transport from the nasal mucosa.

Dr. Schiffman: If aluminum is absorbed into the blood stream, why should it be specifically concentrated in the olfactory areas?

Dr. Edwardson: Because the neurons in those areas, like those in other regions such as the cortex and hippocampus, which selectively accumulate aluminum, appear to be very active metabolically and have very high densities of transferrin receptors.

Dr. Schiffman: Many of our Alzheimer patients have worked in an aluminum-contaminated environment. This is what makes me wonder whether the nasal route is a possibility.

Dr. Edwardson: I agree this should not be ruled out. An important study that may be relevant to this subject was that of Sandra Rifat and her colleagues from Toronto (1). They looked at cognitive impairment in a large group of miners who were deliberately exposed to the inhalation of finely divided aluminum and aluminum oxide to prevent silicosis. They showed clear evidence of cognitive decline in this group and a graded response dependent on the duration of exposure. However, the Toronto group were unable to identify the route of entry of aluminum. It could have got in through the nasal mucosa, but it could also have been swallowed in mucus from the respiratory system and absorbed through the gastrointestinal tract.

Dr. Steen: There is surprisingly similar prevalence of dementia the world over, irrespective of exogenous factors. What range is there in aluminum concentration in the water in different parts of the world?

Dr. Edwardson: I wouldn't suggest for a moment that aluminum is the major environmental risk factor for Alzheimer's disease. It is probably just one among a range of others. Although rates of dementia appear to be relatively uniform globally, neuropathological studies have shown that there is considerable variation in the proportion of patients suffering from multi-infarct dementia compared to Alzheimer's disease, the former being markedly increased in Japan, for example. Overall, Alzheimer's disease accounts for about 50% of all cases of dementia. As far as aluminum in water is concerned, this varies from less than 5 parts per billion in some hard water areas, to 1,000 to 2,000 parts per billion in areas where aluminum treatment is used to remove humic acid and other organic acids. The maximum permitted concentration in the European Community is 200 per billion, but this value is set on practical grounds rather than for any reasons of safety. One possible explanation for the epidemiological data is that it is not the concentration of aluminum that is important but rather the level of silicon, which can vary from 0.5 up to 150 mg per liter.

Dr. Guesry: Is it true that silicon is more abundant in water coming from granitic areas such as Brittany, Cornwall, Scotland, and Ireland? Do you have any information on the rate of Alzheimer's disease in these parts of the world?

Dr. Edwardson: As far as I am aware, granitic rocks are notably resistant to weathering. The very soft waters from these areas cause considerable problems for the water industry because of the content of organic acids, which cause discoloration, and it is these waters particularly that are treated with aluminum. There is much less silicon in these soft waters compared to the amounts present in hard water from the sedimentary rocks. In fact, silicon is often the major solute component of hard water and overall it correlates better with magnesium and calcium than with aluminum.

Dr. Davies: I believe that aluminum-containing antacids are often prescribed for the elderly. Could this be a dangerous prescription in relation to the risk of Alzheimer's disease?

Dr. Edwardson: On the available evidence, it is difficult to say. The question has been examined in a number of epidemiological studies, two of which were large enough to provide adequate data. In one of these no association was found (2); in the other (3), an association was found but it broke down when the analysis examined whether the antacids contained aluminum or not. There is a major problem of informant reliability in retrospective studies and a prospective study is needed. Aluminum absorption is strongly facilitated by acidic conditions and since the prime purpose of giving antacids is to increase gastric pH, the amounts of aluminum absorbed are not nearly so great as one might imagine on the basis of the aluminum ingested. The vast majority of aluminum taken in antacids is simply not absorbed. There is, however, evidence of increased aluminum deposition in bone and soft tissues in people who have taken aluminum-containing antacids over a period of years.

REFERENCES

1. Rifat SL, Eastwood MR, Crapper Mchachlan DR, Corey PN. Effect of exposure of miners to aluminum powder. *Lancet* 1990;336:1162–5.
2. Broe GA, Henderson AS, Creasy H, McCusker E, Korten AE, Jorm AF, Langley W, Anthony JC. A case control study of Alzheimer's disease in Australia. *Neurology* 1990;40:1698–1707.
3. Graves AB, White E, Koepsell TD, Reiffer BV, Van Belle B, Larson EB. The association between aluminum-containing products and Alzheimer's disease. *J Clin Epidemiol* 1990;43:35–44.

Nutrition of the Elderly, edited by H. Munro, and
G. Schlierf, Nestlé Nutrition Workshop Series, Vol. 29,
Nestec Ltd., Vevey/Raven Press, Ltd., New York © 1992.

Practical Aspects of Nutrition of the Elderly at Home

Louise Davies

*Gerontology Nutrition, Royal Free Hospital School of Medicine,
London NW3 2QE, England, UK*

Of the 10 million elderly men and women in the United Kingdom, more than 95% live at home, mostly on their own or with one other person (1). Similarly, in most other countries, developed and developing, the vast majority of old people live in the community. Some manage without undue assistance, others rely on the care of family or support services.

DEFINITION OF ELDERLY

In the United Kingdom the term "elderly" is applied to "persons of pensionable age": women 60 years and over, men 65 years and over. In order to make practical nutritional recommendations there may be advantages in studying the "young old" as a separate group from the "old old," or making a distinction between those who remain independent and those who have become dependent on others (this would be applicable in all countries, whatever the life expectancy).

DIETARY PATTERN

The dietary pattern in the majority of old people remains similar to that established by habits at a younger age and their nutritional status continues to be adequate even in extreme old age (2). Some survive to become "elderly elite"; however, a study in Great Britain reported that malnutrition is likely to be twice as common in the over 80s as in those elderly people under 80 years of age (3). Because of increasing numbers of "old old," there are likely to be greater demands on the already over-stretched social and medical services.

THE ROLE OF PRACTICAL NUTRITION

Practical nutrition for the elderly at home seeks to influence or endorse their food choice in order to help them to achieve and maintain well-being with increasing life expectancy. It has a role in the prevention of malnutrition, in preference to crisis treatment.

TYPES OF MALNUTRITION

Four distinct, but sometimes interrelated, types of malnutrition have been described: specific, sudden, recurrent, and long-standing malnutrition. Each calls for training in recognition and prevention by medical and paramedical personnel, and by care providers, including neighbors and relations (4).

RISK FACTORS

Many studies have identified elderly groups nutritionally at risk of malnutrition through medical, psychological, or socio-economic conditions (5–15). The housebound are one such at-risk group. However, not all housebound people are malnourished, although they might be if, for example, there are circumstances (warning signals) such as insufficient food stores at home or loneliness or observed depression leading to impaired appetite (see Table 1).

WARNING SIGNALS

The concept of observable warning signals has led to the suggestion of a community-based approach to the prevention of malnutrition: care providers in touch with elderly men and women can be taught early recognition of warning signals applicable to their community, and practical steps for simple intervention (16).

Intervention may be simple and inexpensive, for example, help with the shopping, or it may highlight the need for referral for medical or paramedical services, or the

TABLE 1. *Examples of observable warning signals*

Recent unintended weight change ±3 kg
Physical disability affecting food shopping, preparation, or intake
Lack of sunlight
Bereavement and/or observed depression/loneliness
Mental confusion affecting eating
High alcohol consumption
Polypharmacy/long-term medication
Missed meals/snacks/fluids
Food wastage/rejection
Insufficient food stores at home
Lack of fruits/juices/vegetables
Low budget for food
Poor nutritional knowledge

TABLE 2. *Sources of nutritional knowledge*

	%
Newspapers/magazines	83
Books	69
Television	69
Radio	60
Relations	53
Food labels	40
Doctor	10

urgency for introduction to a total package of care, including meals programs or other community services.

PRACTICAL NUTRITION FOR THE "YOUNG OLD"

Prevention of malnutrition in elderly people begins with the "young old" and dietary guidelines have taken their rightful place in the forefront of preventive medicine. Despite this, investigations on men and women around the time of retirement from work have revealed, for example, fat intakes markedly higher than current recommendations (17). At retirement, there is motivation to maintain health and independence, but this is hampered by confusion with the multiplicity of messages and lack of guidance from the medical profession (18), as indicated in Table 2. Nutritional guidance is needed for conditions that could interfere with preparation and enjoyment of food; these include increasingly reported joint and muscle pains, impaired hearing, anxieties, depression and stress, lack of exercise, dependence on medication, and smoking. Unfortunately, practical nutrition rarely forms a part of medical training. This stresses the importance of the dietitian.

Perhaps the most important message practical nutrition can give to the "young old" is one of moderation.

PRACTICAL NUTRITION FOR THE "OLD OLD"

For the "old old" remaining relatively healthy and independent at home, the question that needs to be asked is not "can we alter food habits?," but rather "should we?". By the time men and women have survived to advanced old age, the dietary risks are lessened. Lowering salt and sugar reduces palatability, and restricting fat reduces energy and nutrient intakes and diminishes palatability. For elderly individuals, it is important to keep up the enjoyment of food and not to be overrestrictive.

NUTRITIONAL COUNSELING

Counseling may be needed on, for example, obesity, exercise, sunlight, drug–nutrient interactions, supplements versus foods, dietary fiber, and fluids. Practical advice can reach elderly men and women through specialized cookbooks, shopping checklists, talks and demonstrations in clubs, retirement cookery classes, and informative, entertaining programs on radio and television.

CONTRIBUTION BY THE FOOD INDUSTRY

It is not true that "the elderly are set in their ways and will not try new foods." Food manufacturers and shopkeepers—and nutrition educators—would do well to note the major influences on change in food choice among elderly men and women: health, taste, convenience, price, and availability in small portions (19).

The food industry can assist this choice by producing enjoyable, nourishing, easy to prepare foods; easy to open and store; available in small sizes at reasonable cost; a changing variety of small packs of nutritious instant and convenience foods. Foods need to be nutrient-dense, especially for those with diminished appetite, giving maximum nourishment and maximum safety with minimum effort. They also need to take into account maximum acceptability in flavor, texture, aroma, and appearance.

PRACTICAL NUTRITION FOR THE FRAIL ELDERLY

Without adequate nutritional and social support, old people may need to be placed too early into total care. With adequate nutrition, they may achieve a greater resistance to disease and speedier recovery from illness. Negative stereotypes need to be questioned, for example, "they eat less as they grow older"; "they need soft/ pureed foods because they cannot chew"; "they need dietary supplements." These may apply to some, but certainly not to all.

PRACTICAL NUTRITION FOR AND FROM THE CARE PROVIDERS

It may be necessary to provide old people with extra help for shopping and food preparation; for some, assistive feeding equipment and adaptations to the kitchen can encourage self-help.

It is advisable to provide nutritional guidance not only to the old people themselves but also to those who may be caring for them in the community. This may include recipe guidance for those providing meals at home, delivered meals, or meals at clubs or day hospitals.

MEALS PROGRAMS

Meals programs need to be seen in the context of the total diet. In the United Kingdom there have been imaginative alternatives suggested to meals on wheels, for example, small freezers, microwaves or steamers provided in the client's home, and suitable meals delivered in batches so that they can be chosen and cooked at the time most desired by the old person. Food policies have been established. Their aim is to provide food within a prescribed budget that is nutritionally sound, safe to eat, looks attractive, tastes good, and is enjoyed by the clients. Enjoyment of food is paramount (20).

It must be remembered that food that is not eaten is not nourishing.

REFERENCES

1. Population figures. Sources: Office of Population Censuses and Surveys; General Register Office (Scotland); General Register Office (Northern Ireland).
2. Exton-Smith AN. Nutritional status: diagnosis and prevention of malnutrition. In: Exton-Smith AN, Caird FI, eds. *Metabolic and nutritional disorders in the elderly.* Bristol: John Wright, 1980:66–76.
3. Department of Health and Social Security. *Nutrition and health in old age.* Reports on Health and Social Subjects No 16. London: HMSO, 1979.
4. Davies L. Practical nutrition for the elderly. *Nutr Rev* 1988;46:83–7.
5. Tomaiolo PP. Malnutrition in the elderly: its recognition and treatment. *Compr Ther* 1985;11:54–8.
6. Hanson BS, Mattisson I, Steen B. Dietary intake and psychosocial factors in 68-year-old men: a population study. *Compr Gerontol (B)* 1987;1:62–7.
7. Steen B, Isaksson B, Svanborg A. Intake of energy and nutrients and meal habits in 70-year old males and females in Gothenburg, Sweden: a population study. *Acta Med Scand* 1977;611(suppl): 39–86.
8. Colucci RA, Bell SJ, Blackburn GL. Nutritional problems of institutionalized and free-living elderly. *Compr Ther* 1987;13:20–8.
9. Morley JE. Nutritional problems in the elderly. *Contemp Nutr* 1987;12:1.
10. McIntosh WA, Shifflett PA, Picou JS. Social support, stressful events, strain, dietary intake, and the elderly. *Med Care* 1989;27:140–53.
11. Horwath CC. Marriage and diet in elderly Australians: results from a large random survey. *J Hum Nutr Diet* 1989;2:185–93.
12. Horwath CC. Socio-economic status and dietary habits in the elderly: results from a large random survey. *J Hum Nutr Diet* 1989;2:173–83.
13. Sem SW, Nes M, Engeldal K, Pedersen JI, Trygg K. An attempt to identify and describe a group of non-institutionalised elderly with the lowest nutrient score. *Compr Gerontol (A)* 1988;2:60–6.
14. Cashman MD, Wightkin WT. Geriatric malnutrition: recognition and prevention. *Compr Ther* 1987;13:45–51.
15. Roe DA. Drug-induced malnutrition in geriatric patients. *Compr Ther* 1977;3:24–8.
16. Davies L, Knutson KC. Warning signals for malnutrition in the elderly. *J Am Diet Assoc* 1991;11:1413–17.
17. Committee on Medical Aspects of Food Policy (COMA). *Diet and cardiovascular disease.* Reports on Health and Social Subjects No 28. London: DHSS, 1984.
18. Davies L, Anderson JP, Holdsworth MD. Nutrition education at the age of retirement from work. *Health Educ J* 1985;44:187–92.
19. Bilderbeck N, Holdsworth MD, Purves R, Davies L. Changing food habits among 100 elderly men and women in the United Kingdom. *J Hum Nutr* 1981;35:448–55.
20. Davies L. Opportunities for better health in the elderly through mass catering. A document of the Nutrition Unit, World Health Organization, Regional Office for Europe, Copenhagen, Denmark (in press).

DISCUSSION

Dr. Meredith: How do you deal with fadism in the older age group? I have seen people who put soy protein powder on everything because they think they are protein deficient.

Dr. Davies: This is where the medical profession can help enormously. People have food beliefs that sometimes don't matter, but sometimes they do, and what the doctor says is usually believed. The doctor should provide an opportunity for discussing diet and food beliefs.

Dr. Vellas: One characteristic of elderly people is that weight lost after stress is often not regained. How do you explain this?

Dr. Davies: Failure to regain weight loss could of course be due to disease. It could also be due to factors such as loneliness, which may inhibit eating. This is where our warning signal concept is useful. One of the warning signals is weight change. This should trigger an investigation into possible social or disease factors.

Dr. Vellas: I should like to make a comment on malnutrition in the elderly based on the Aging Process Study in New Mexico. This is a longitudinal study of 200 elderly people in good health. Between 1980, when the mean age was 72 years, and 1990 there has been no decrease in average weight in this population nor in arm circumference. There has been a small *increase* in serum albumin. Thus, the aging process alone is not a cause of malnutrition in this population. There are three patterns of malnutrition in this age group. First, there is disease such as malignancy or Alzheimer's disease; then there is acute disease such as a stroke or a fracture; and finally there is malnutrition associated with the normal aging process. In order to prevent malnutrition in the elderly population it is very important to measure weight and to do diagnostic investigations if there is weight loss. The earlier a problem is recognized, the more chance there will be of sorting it out and preventing the development of serious malnutrition.

Dr. Guesry: For a company like ours, it is tempting to develop products for the elderly specially adapted to their needs in terms of taste, texture, packaging, nutritional content, and so on. The big problem is that the elderly don't want to be told they are old, so I think such products are likely to remain on the shelves. What is your view of this marketing problem?

Dr. Davies: I faced this some years ago when I wrote a book called *Easy Cooking for One or Two.* There was no mention of the elderly in the title for precisely this reason, but I deliberately chose foods that I knew old people like and I made them as nourishing and tempting as possible, and in small quantities because a lot of old people do not want to buy food and waste it. What I think is needed is nice flavor and suitably small packaging. I have tasted many of the foods put on the market for the elderly and there is no way I should want to continue to eat them! If you were to produce nourishing, good tasting food in small quantities, I think the problem would be solved.

Dr. Steen: How do you think the responsibility for old people should be divided between the various agencies?

Dr. Davies: In the first place, it is clear that a majority of old people would prefer to look after themselves with the help of relatives, friends, and neighbors. This is not always possible and there are cases where the social services have to be involved. But there should not be a lot of government officials making independent inquiries. It is far preferable to have one care worker, with access to the provision of a variety of services, responsible for evaluating the needs and wishes of the old person. What is happening in Britain at the moment is that, because of limited funds and services, there has been a devolution of responsibility away from social services and into the private sector. This has advantages but it also has dangers, particularly from the point of view of cost for old people.

Dr. Steen: The reason I asked my question was that I am concerned that some countries pay more attention to the needs of healthy elderly people than they do to providing diagnosis, therapy, and rehabilitation for really ill people.

Dr. Davies: Of course, diagnosis, therapy, and rehabilitation are important, but by paying attention to the needs of healthy elderly people (including their socio-economic and psychological needs), we can often provide sufficient support, including incentive for self-help, to prevent the health crisis. I think what you are talking about is balance of provision, so that limited resources are not squandered. As I implied in my previous answer, holistic assessment (for therapeutic and social goals) is essential to ensure that provision of service is targeted to individual needs. Without this assessment there is the risk of providing some people with more help than they need while denying others sufficient help. Holistic assessment of old people in whom subclinical malnutrition might be prevented must surely be preferable to crisis treatment, both in human and financial terms.

Dr. Schiffman: What are your thoughts about texture preferences of older people? How much energy are they willing to put into chewing and crunching? Do they like grainy foods or crunchy foods? What is your impression of the British population?

Dr. Davies: Most old people like food to have texture. In fact, it is observed that, when offered attractive food that is difficult to chew, they will often remove their dentures and masticate the food with their hard gums. However, they are inclined to avoid food that works its way painfully under dentures, or that may cause choking, for example, fruits with pips and fish with small bones. A pureed diet should be offered only for short-term necessity, with re-evaluation for a return as soon as possible to food with texture. In rehabilitation it is important for people to be encouraged to use their chewing ability.

Nutrition of the Elderly, edited by H. Munro, and
G. Schlierf, Nestlé Nutrition Workshop Series, Vol. 29,
Nestec Ltd., Vevey/Raven Press, Ltd., New York © 1992.

Practical Aspects of Nutrition of the Elderly in Institutions

Bertil Steen

*Department of Geriatric Medicine, Gothenburg University,
Gothenburg, Sweden*

Although most studies of elderly populations living at home in countries like Sweden show on average acceptable dietary habits compared to the rest of the population, at least up to the age of 80 years, even though variation may be considerable (1–5), the situation may be quite different when the elderly come to institutions and are forced to live there for medical and/or social reasons. There are many reasons for this, most relating to the fact that such elderly people are older, more frail, and suffering from a variety of often serious diseases. However, factors relating to the hospital or nursing home environment are also relevant.

Even before admission to institutions, risk factors and practical aspects relating to nutrition at home, as reviewed, for example, by Davies (6), are of obvious relevance to the institutional nutritional situation. Low intakes of energy and nutrients have been reported from institutions in several countries, such as Denmark (7), Sweden (8,9), the United Kingdom (10), and the United States (11). Some of these patients have been said to suffer from "hospital malnutrition" (12). It has been clearly shown that the undernourished do worse than the well nourished in regard to serious complications and mortality (13,14).

There are many possible causes of malnutrition in institutions (Table 1). For a review, see ref. 15. Some of these will be dealt with below.

DISEASE *PER SE*

Obstacles to proper feeding in institutionalized elderly people include poor appetite, anorexia, and vomiting due to disease. Physical and mental handicap, such

TABLE 1. *Factors that may affect the nutritional situation in institutions*

Disease *per se*	Meal environment
Oral health	Meal distribution through the day
Dehydration	Knowledge and understanding among the staff
Drug treatment	Nutritional supplement policy
Physical activity	Terminal phase of life

211

as stroke, parkinsonism, rheumatoid arthritis, depression, confusion, and dementia may all interfere with eating. In certain groups, such as demented and psychotic patients (16) and somatic long-term care patients (17), the prevalence of "hospital malnutrition" can be very high—20% to 35%, and 15% to 25%, respectively.

A practical problem in giving patients nutritional advice is presented by different degrees of hearing loss. In one study in elderly nursing home patients (18), all patients tested had considerably impaired hearing. Mean hearing loss in the speech area was 51 dB, indicating that the majority of the patients needed hearing aids. However, only 1 patient in 10 had one, and technical devices for amplification in the wards were scarce. It was evident that impaired hearing among these patients was an underestimated and rather neglected problem.

As mentioned, severe nutritional problems may result from confusional states and dementia. In depression, loss of appetite and malnutrition are often diagnostic and at the same time are a difficult therapeutic problem. Indeed, one of the most difficult situations in geriatric medicine is to decide if food refusal is due to curable depression or a voluntary desire to give up in a mentally healthy individual.

DEHYDRATION

Water is of course essential for all biological functions in the body. Since water is lost in many common conditions in institutions, such as diarrhea, fever, and renal diseases, the risk of dehydration in such elderly patients is obvious (19). It has also been shown that elderly people seem to experience less thirst than younger people in water deficit (20), and renal concentrating ability is also less (21). The risk may be further aggravated by frequent treatment with diuretic drugs. It has also been shown that the decrease of body weight during the eighth decade of life is mostly related to a decreasing amount of body water, especially extracellular water (22). In certain institutionalized elderly people at risk it may for these reasons be practical to prescribe water as a drug—"one large glass of water four times daily."

ORAL HEALTH

Despite the fact that the population of elderly people at large seem to have better oral health now than just a few decades ago, at least in countries like Sweden (23), this is not true to the same degree regarding elderly patients in institutions. Data concerning the relation between dental state and dietary intake are not conclusive. There are also many confounding factors (24), such as socioeconomic and psychological factors, and the use or misuse of alcohol or tobacco. There are no clear-cut data to support the hypothesis that natural dentition is necessary for elderly people to maintain a satisfactory nutritional state. However, there seems to be a relation between poor dental state and difficulties of ingesting certain food items, such as meat and hard foods (25). Easily chewed food items may also predispose to dryness of the mouth, which may be enhanced by drug treatment. Several oral and dental

conditions, such as angular stomatitis, denture stomatitis, glossitis, and bone resorption may be related to poor eating habits or inadequate diet, and atrophy of the
oral mucosa may also be caused by poor oral hygiene and faulty dentures.

DRUG TREATMENT

Drug treatment may give rise to poor appetite and/or vomiting, the best known
example being digitalis treatment. The commonly used treatment with diuretic drugs
enhances the danger of dehydration, and treatment with diuretic or psychotropic
drugs may also cause dryness of the mouth, which makes chewing and eating still
more difficult.

PHYSICAL ACTIVITY

Many institutionalized elderly patients are physically inactive, which gives rise to
low needs for energy and therefore difficulties in maintaining a sufficient intake of
essential nutrients. Furthermore, physical inactivity enhances bone mineral losses
from the skeleton, and several studies have shown that exercise can prevent or
reverse some of the limiting changes in cardiovascular function and work capacity
and be able to improve glucose tolerance (for review, see ref. 26).

MEAL ENVIRONMENT

An unsuitable meal environment is an important negative factor in institutional
nutrition. In one study an improved meal environment in a nursing home was studied
(17). The dining room of the nursing home was changed from a very sterile environment to an environment typical of the 1940s when these patients had their most
active period. Prior to the change the measured average energy intake was very low,
and, as an example of nutrients, the average intake of vitamin D was only 2.8 Mg.
The dietary intake improved significantly during the experimental period, and the
intakes of energy and protein increased by 25%. Physical activity increased as well,
and the psychological evaluation showed improvements in conversation, facial
expression, and social interest.

MEAL DISTRIBUTION THROUGH THE DAY

An improper distribution of meals may be disadvantageous. The recommendations
in Sweden suggest three major meals and two in-between snacks during the day in
hospitals and nursing homes. However, this is not always the case, and sometimes
three or four meals can be served during about 8 hours followed by as much as 16
hours of overnight starvation. It is obvious that the appetite may be very poor during

these meals when they are so close. For a review of these problems and details of studies concerning meal distribution, see ref. 27.

KNOWLEDGE AND UNDERSTANDING AMONG THE STAFF

Insufficient knowledge and understanding of nutritional problems among the hospital or nursing home staff, including doctors, are important causes of insufficient nutrition. The need for education and training is obvious. One method for improvement is the appointment of one nurse in every ward to be responsible for the nutrition in that particular ward, and thus be a link between the ward, the physicians, the dietitians, and the hospital kitchen.

NUTRITIONAL SUPPLEMENT POLICY

Doctors and nurses may sometimes not be aware of the improvements that may be achieved by use of dietary supplements. As an example can be mentioned a study in a somatic nursing home, where three different kinds of dietary supplements were given during an experimental period (28). Before the study the energy intakes were low, on average 1,247 kcal. During the experimental period the intake of energy increased by 25%. The decrease in appetite at the main meals caused by the supplementation was very low, whereas the intakes of less valuable in-between meals decreased from 20% to 11% of the energy intake.

TERMINAL PHASE OF LIFE

Nutrition is a prominent problem among the many ethical and medical problems in the terminal phase of life. Ethicists are discussing these problems in terms of the concept of sanctity of life as opposed to quality of life (29,30), there being a general trend for the former gradually to be replaced by the latter. These problems have also been discussed from a religious point of view, for example, in relation to Judaism (31) and to Catholicism (32).

Indications for fluid therapy as well the subject of thirst sensation in the last phase of life have been extensively discussed (for a review, see ref. 33). However, no clear-cut recommendations can be established from currently available publications.

CONCLUSION

In this chapter some possible causes of "hospital malnutrition" have been described. Some may be dealt with, others not. The most important thing is to be aware of the problems. After that, solutions are often possible in hospitals and nursing homes.

REFERENCES

1. Steen B, Isaksson B, Svanborg A. Intake of energy and nutrients and meal habits in 70-year-old males and females in Gothenburg, Sweden. A population study. *Acta Med Scand* 1977;611(suppl): 39–86.
2. Lundgren BK, Steen B, Isaksson B. Dietary habits in 70- and 75-year old males and females. Longitudinal and cohort data from a population study. *Näringsforskning* 1987;31:53–6.
3. Nordström G, Lundgren BK, Nilsson B, Steen B, Österlind P-O. Dietary habits in the eighth decade of life. *Compr Gerontol* 1988;A2:29–39.
4. Hanson BS, Mattisson I, Steen B. Dietary intake and psychosocial factors in 68-year-old men. A population study. *Compr Gerontol* 1987;B1:62–7.
5. Steen B, Nilsson K, Robertsson E, Östberg H. Age retirement in women. II. Dietary habits and body composition. *Compr Gerontol* 1988;A2:78–82.
6. Davies L. Socioeconomic, psychosocial and educational aspects of nutrition in old age. *Age Ageing* 1990;19(suppl 1):S37–42.
7. Hessov I. Energy and protein intake in elderly patients in an orthopedic surgical ward. *Acta Chir Scand* 1977;143:145–9.
8. Steen B. Intake of protein in geriatric long-term patients. *Aktuel Gerontol* 1980;10:515–9.
9. Elmståhl S, Steen B. Hospital nutrition in geriatric long-term care medicine. II. Effects of dietary supplements. *Age Ageing* 1987;16:73–80.
10. Hachet AF, Yeung CK, Hill GL. Eating patterns in patients recovering from major surgery—a study of voluntary food intake and energy balance. *Br J Surg* 1979;66:415–9.
11. Steffee WP. Malnutrition in hospitalized patients. *JAMA* 1980;244:2630–5.
12. Blackburn GL, Butterworth C. Hospital malnutrition. *Nutrition Today* 1975;3:8–18.
13. Linn BS. Outcomes of older and younger malnourished and wellnourished patients one year after hospitalization. *Am J Clin Nutr* 1984;39:66–73.
14. Warnold I, Lundholm K. Clinical significance of preoperative nutritional status in 215 non-cancer patients. *Ann Surg* 1984;199:299–305.
15. Steen B. Causes, prevention, and treatment of hospital malnutrition. In: Watson RR, ed. *Nutrition and heart disease*, vol II. Boca Raton, FL: CRC Press, 1987:83–8.
16. Asplund K, Normark M, Pettersson V. Nutritional assessment of psychogeriatric patients. *Age Ageing* 1981;10:87–94.
17. Elmståhl S, Blabolil V, Fex G, Küller R, Steen B. Hospital nutrition in geriatric long-term care medicine. I. Effects of a changed meal environment. *Compr Gerontol* 1987;A1:29–33.
18. Hedner K, Broms P, Harris S, Steen B. Hearing in geriatric long-stay patients. *Compr Gerontol* 1987;A1:69–71.
19. Massler M. Geriatric nutrition 11: Dehydration in the elderly. *J Prosthet Dent* 1979;42:489–91.
20. Phillips PA, Rolls BJ, Ledingham JGG, et al. Reduced thirst after water deprivation in healthy elderly men. *N Engl J Med* 1984;311:753–9.
21. Lindeman RD. Van Buren HC, Raisz LG. Osmolar renal concentration ability in healthy young men and hospitalized patients without renal disease. *N Engl J Med* 1960;262:1306–9.
22. Steen B, Lundgren BK, Isaksson B. Body composition at age 70, 75, 79 and 81. A longitudinal population study. In: Chandra RK, ed. *Nutrition, immunity and illness in the elderly*. Exeter, UK: Pergamon Press, 1985:49–52.
23. Österberg T, Mellström D. Tobacco smoking: a major risk factor for loss of teeth in three 70-year-old cohorts. *Community Dent Oral Epidemiol* 1986;14:367–70.
24. Heath MR. Dietary selection by elderly persons, related to dental state. *Br Dent J* 1972;132:145–8.
25. Österberg T, Steen B. Relationship between dental state and dietary intake in 70-year-old males and females in Göteborg, Sweden. A population study. *J Oral Rehab* 1982;9:509–21.
26. Smith EL, Smith PE, Gilligan C. Diet, exercise, and chronic disease pattern in older adults. *Nutr Rev* 1988;46:52–61.
27. Isaksson B. How to avoid malnutrition during hospitalization? *Hum Nutr Appl Nutr* 1982;36A: 367–70.
28. Elmståhl S, Steen B. Hospital nutrition in geriatric long-term care medicine. II. Effects of dietary supplements. *Age Ageing* 1987;16:73–80.
29. Levinson AR. Termination of life support systems in the elderly. Ethical issues. *J Geriatr Psychiatry* 1981;14:71–9.

30. Robertson GS. Dealing with the brain-damaged old—dignity before sanctity. *J Med Ethics* 1982;8: 173–6.
31. Bleich JD. The Quinlan case: a Jewish perspective. In: Rossner F, Bleich JD, eds. *Jewish bioethics.* New York: Sanhedrin Press, 1979.
32. Pope Pius XII. The prolongation of life. *The Pope speaks.* 1958;4:393.
33. Michaelsson E, Norberg A, Norberg B. Feeding methods for demented patients in end stage of life. *Geriatr Nursing* 1987;8:69–73.

DISCUSSION

Dr. Hodkinson: A nursing colleague looked at institutional starvation in our own facility in the long stay wards. She found some interesting things. One of the real problems about adequate feeding of these patients is pressure of time. The feeding of helpless old people occupies an enormous amount of nursing effort, yet institutional rules limit time quite severely because of the rigidity of the routines. One of the particular markers of poor nutrition in patients who eat slowly is a rigid kitchen routine. The other thing she found was that the nursing staff were not very good at recognizing which patients were at greatest nutritional risk. The ones they identified as being at risk were often the ones with strange dietary habits, but measurements showed that their intakes were generally quite high. Other patients about whom the staff were not so worried were the slow eaters and these often had very poor intakes. There is thus a need for better education of the nursing staff and a need to develop strategies to encourage old people to eat, and even to eat more quickly.

Dr. Steen: A crucial problem is to make all medical staff aware of the fact that nutrition is a very important part of medicine, as important as drug therapy, surgery, or physiotherapy. What we started to do 15 years ago was to ensure that on every geriatric ward there is a nurse who has special responsibility for nutrition. These nurses are given a 30-hour course on basic nutrition. They have responsibility for being the link between the kitchens, the doctors, the ward, and the patients.

Dr. Hodkinson: Another difficulty is the nutrient density. This is particularly the case when patients with feeding difficulties are given pureed foods. The nutrient density of such foods is often extremely low. It could easily be increased by the addition of complex polysaccharides without altering the taste too much. I think this simple practice has been neglected. It would be very easy to do.

Dr. Steen: I agree completely. In some patients the need is for energy rather than for protein or other nutrients. Professor Munro has shown that at very low energy intakes, energy is more important than protein in obtaining a positive nitrogen balance.

Dr. Davies: I recognize that in the elderly with disease states, the provision of supplements is often necessary, but I wonder whether sometimes it is done just for convenience. It is easier to give a vitamin C pill than to provide a nice fruit salad and wait for it to be eaten, for example. There is often a danger that the convenience of staff is placed first to the detriment of the resident old people. We always tell our staff: you know your slow eaters so why don't you serve them first and clear their table last. This makes quite a difference in time and is just common sense.

Dr. Steen: I agree this is the ideal. However, I think that dietary supplements, and I don't mean vitamins but nutritional supplements, are of value in institutions and in elderly people's own homes. In a study in which we gave 500 kcal by supplement, the energy intake increased by 25%, with practically no decrease in appetite for the main meals.

Dr. Edwardson: People who administer institutions caring for the elderly must be more flexible. The vast majority of institutions that I know of discourage families and visitors at meal times, whereas in terms of support meal times would be very suitable visiting times, since relatives could give valuable assistance with feeding.

Dr. Vellas: One problem is that it is very difficult to feed sick elderly patients with anorexia who don't want to eat.

Dr. Doyle: One of the strategies that we are using to help solve this feeding problem is to recruit and train retired nurses living in a retirement community. Dietitians and nurses together train these people on the methodology of correct feeding and it seems to be working. We also encourage family members to come in and some have been trained as well.

Nutrition of the Elderly, edited by H. Munro, and
G. Schlierf, Nestlé Nutrition Workshop Series, Vol. 29,
Nestec Ltd., Vevey/Raven Press, Ltd., New York © 1992.

Concluding Remarks

Günter Schlierf

*Department of Medicine/Geriatrics, Bethanien Hospital Heidelberg,
6900 Heidelberg 1, Germany*

In concluding rather than summarizing this interesting meeting, I would like to make three points and present three tables.

An American born today has a good chance of still being alive in 2062. In order to expect fair health one must, among other things, carefully watch one's diet. In contrast to those who sailed across the ocean to discover this country and as a rule did not live long enough to experience either myocardial infarction or osteoporosis, we and our children have to try to ensure that our organs, from brain and teeth to bowels and feet, will last in function for 80 rather than 40 years. So, one most important issue for nutrition and the elderly concerns the decades *before* we are old. We have learned a lot during this meeting, which relates to prolongation of the disease-free life expectancy, which is what we should aim for.

A second point relates to nutrition *during* old age. In dealing with nutritional requirements of the elderly we must be impressed by the great heterogeneity of this group. We need to consider at least three categories, namely, the elderly, the old, and the very old. If a man of 69 or a woman of 73, in addition to having good genes, has eaten sensibly and been physically active, he or she will show few if any of the changes in body composition that have been discussed in this volume. If we continue to eat a prudent, balanced diet, even if we are 80 or above, nutritionists will still not find evidence of malnutrition.

My third and final point then relates to the very old and sick, and we have seen that there are many. Here we find malnutrition and here we encounter numerous unresolved questions regarding requirements, as affected by diseases and their treatments, and how those requirements can be met. Tables 1 to 3, taken from a study

TABLE 1. *BEST-study: vitamin status*

Satisfactory	33%
One vitamin "deficient"	36%
Two vitamins "deficient"	15%
Three vitamins "deficient"	9%
Four vitamins "deficient"	6%

From Platt D(1).

TABLE 2. *Vitamin status of elderly people: frequency of values outside conventional limits*

	Healthy elderly (>65 years) (%)	Geriatric patients (>75 years) (%)
Vitamin A	7	43
Vitamin C	8	26
Vitamin B_1—αETK^a	3	15
Vitamin B_2—αEGR^a	4	20
Vitamin B_6—$\alpha EGOT^a$	8	14

[a] Enzyme assays from (1).

on nutritional status in a random sample of very old patients admitted to hospital, show a high frequency of unsatisfactory vitamin status and very poor nutrient intakes, when compared to intakes recommended by the German Nutrition Society. It is evident that a lot needs to be done in this area. It is with the sick and the very old that we experience our limitations.

TABLE 3. *Median nutrient intake [24-hr recall in women (n = 69) and men (n = 25)]*

	Women		Men	
	Intake	DGE recom	Intake	DGE recom
Energy (kcal)	1533	1700	1678	1900
Protein (g)	55	45	62	55
Fat (g)	66	<55	73	<61
Carbohydrate (g)	158		172	
Alcohol (g)	0.02		5	
Fiber (g)	13		15	
Purine (mg)	310		448	
Cholesterol (mg)	220		300	
Na (mg)	1504		2174	
K (mg)	2208	3500	2095	3500
Mg (mg)	184	300	196	350
Ca (mg)	445	800	454	800
Fe (mg)	10	12	12	12
P (mg)	873	800	969	800
Retinol (mg)	0.51	0.8	0.66	1.0
Vit. D (µg)	1.29	5	1.32	5
Vit. E (mg)	7.64	12	7.76	12
Folate (µg)	143.96	160	136.10	160
Vitamin B_1 (mg)	0.97	1.1	0.98	1.3
Vitamin B_2 (mg)	1.02	1.5	0.99	1.7
Vitamin B_6 (mg)	1.21	1.6	1.35	1.8
Vitamin C (mg)	102.02	75	57.84	75

DGE recom: Recommendations of the German Nutrition Society.
From Platt D(1).

We have learned a lot from this conference—of things we should know and of those we do not yet know. On behalf of all, I would like to thank the speakers for sharing with us the fruits of their work and Dr. Guesry and his staff for giving them and us this opportunity.

REFERENCE

1. Platt D, Gerontology. In: Schlierf G, Volkert D, Frauenrath C, et al. *Nutritional Problems in Geriatric Patients*, Springer-Verlag, 1989;213–20.
2. Gerontology, 4th International Symposium. Platt D, ed. *Present state and research perspectives in the experimental and clinical gerontology*. Heidelberg: Springer, 1989.

Subject Index